IDEAL WEIGHTS

Attaining Your Ideal While Achieving Lasting Success—Even Post Menopause!

Dr. Mahnaz Entezami Azim-Zadeh (also known as Dr. Azim)

First Edition, 2020

ISBN 978-0-578-72309-9

Editor: Katheirne Factor

Book Design: Alison Nordin

Consultant: Niki Azim

IDEAL WEIGHTS

Attaining Your Ideal While Achieving Lasting Success—Even Post Menopause!

DR. MAHNAZ AZIM, DOCTOR OF CHIROPRACTIC

Health and Nutrition Coach, IIN | Bioidentical Hormone Replacement Therapist, AMA | Fitness Nutrition Specialist, NASM | Personal Trainer, NASM

DISCLAIMER: The contents of this book are not intended to replace direct supervision by your physician. Although every effort has been made to gather the correct information to support your wellness journey, medicine is a science of constant change and physicians have different theories and approaches to treating a variety of medical and health issues. This book simply offers an additional path to maintain a healthier lifestyle. The advice provided herein should be performed or used in conjunction with clearance from your physician or healthcare provider.

Dr. Mahnaz Entezami Azim-Zadeh, DC, will not be held liable from potential risks arising from any and all contents listed in this book, which include but are not limited to food selection(s), dietary habit(s), exercise technique(s) and/or wellness and self-care suggestions, etc. Any and all contents of this book are not meant for all person(s) and said person(s) are strongly recommended to use said contents in addition to physician-assisted guidance. Thus, all person(s) assume responsibility for any possible risk(s), which may occur from following any and all content available in this book.

DEDICATION

This book is for my parents, whose selfless acts allowed me to follow my dreams. It is also for my brothers. To my youngest brother, Afshin, a brilliant young man that lost his life fighting for his country; Mansour, who has been my confidante keeping me focused on what is important; and for my oldest brother, Massoud, who lost his life after a long battle with a brain injury. Massoud's dedication and effort helped me in my journey from Iran to the United States. My family is never far from my heart.

And last but not least, I want to dedicate this labor of love to my caring and hard-working children. To my darling daughter Niki, who is a juris doctor; and to my loving son, Ari, who is an entrepreneur.

FOREWORD

SINCE BECOMING AN ALTERNATIVE CARE provider in 1996, my goal has remained the same: to provide the highest standard in quality healthcare through coaching clients in healthy lifestyles, while maintaining a positive spirit and furthering my knowledge and education.

MY JOURNEY TO HELP YOU toward ideal health began in my youth. I was born and raised as one of seven children in western Iran. My mom had her hands full with all seven of us, but whenever we got sick, she was quick to make us feel better. It seems like just yesterday that she would take us to see the medical doctor about whatever ailed us. Then we would head to the town's herbalist and watch her compound our healing concoctions. That's what I knew medicine to be—a natural solution whenever possible.

In 1978, I moved to the United States to pursue my studies in alternative healthcare. After passing my first hurdle—learning English as a second language—I went on to receive my Bachelor's Degree of Science in Biology from Portland State University and pursue the healthcare path for years to come.

DRAWN TO THE INTRICACIES OF THE BODY and anatomy, I was especially in awe of how the spine and nervous system are connected to every aspect of the body, and therefore so important to overall health. I decided to become a chiropractor and returned to school at the Cleveland Chiropractic College in Los Angeles. I then became a certified Spinal Biomechanics Specialist from the Pettibon Institute, giving me a wealth of knowledge about the spine.

I found myself having a constant curiosity tied to discovering how the body worked optimally. I noticed too many patients in pain, caught in crash diet roller coasters, engaging in constant self-criticism, or stalled on goals. I soon realized that my overweight and obese patients with lower back and knee pain felt a lot better after losing as little as 5–10 pounds.

Observing such progress inspired me to dig into nutrition and the modalities that could support them even better. I became a certified Fitness Nutrition Specialist, a certified Health and Nutrition Coach, a Personal Trainer, a Corrective Exercise Specialist, and a Weight Loss Specialist. I am also a certified Bioidentical Hormone Replacement Therapist—I want to help women in transition!

WHAT INSPIRED *IDEAL WEIGHTS*? Well, after years of applying my education and knowledge to my clients, I saw fluctuating dietary patterns differed from client to client based on age, weight, height, and other personal factors. Because personal factors differ, it became increasingly difficult to find a single solution for all of my clients, but even more challenging was the maintenance of such weight loss. There wasn't *one* ideal outcome or weight range, there were *many*.

This experience led me to investigate the importance of Ideal Weights as a holistic program. In this book, you will find surefire methods that—if followed and maintained—can lead to lasting success in weight loss.

I TRULY LOVE SHARING MY INSIGHT that arises from my personal and my patients' results. When using the Ideal Weights approach properly, you may achieve positive changes and sustain said changes under your own terms.

When I see positive changes in a patient's blood tests that then cause their doctors to take them off medications, I'm having a good day. There is nothing better than watching clients close in on an ideal weight. But also, I help them feel better, reverse type 2 diabetes or fatty liver disease, lower blood sugar or blood pressure or their LDL (bad cholesterol). Not only have I seen the wonderfully vital lifestyle affect others, but this path has also made *me* stronger, more fit, and—best of all—happier, so I can better serve you.

I've dedicated my coaching to helping you create realistic goals for healthy living with lasting results. I am here for you!

YOURS IN HEALTH,

DR. MAHNAZ AZIM, DC

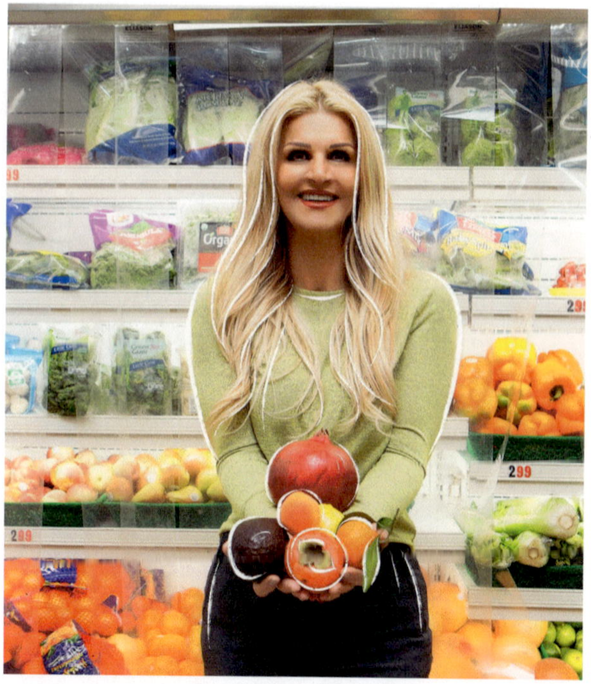

"Natural forces within us are the true healers of disease."

-Hippocrates

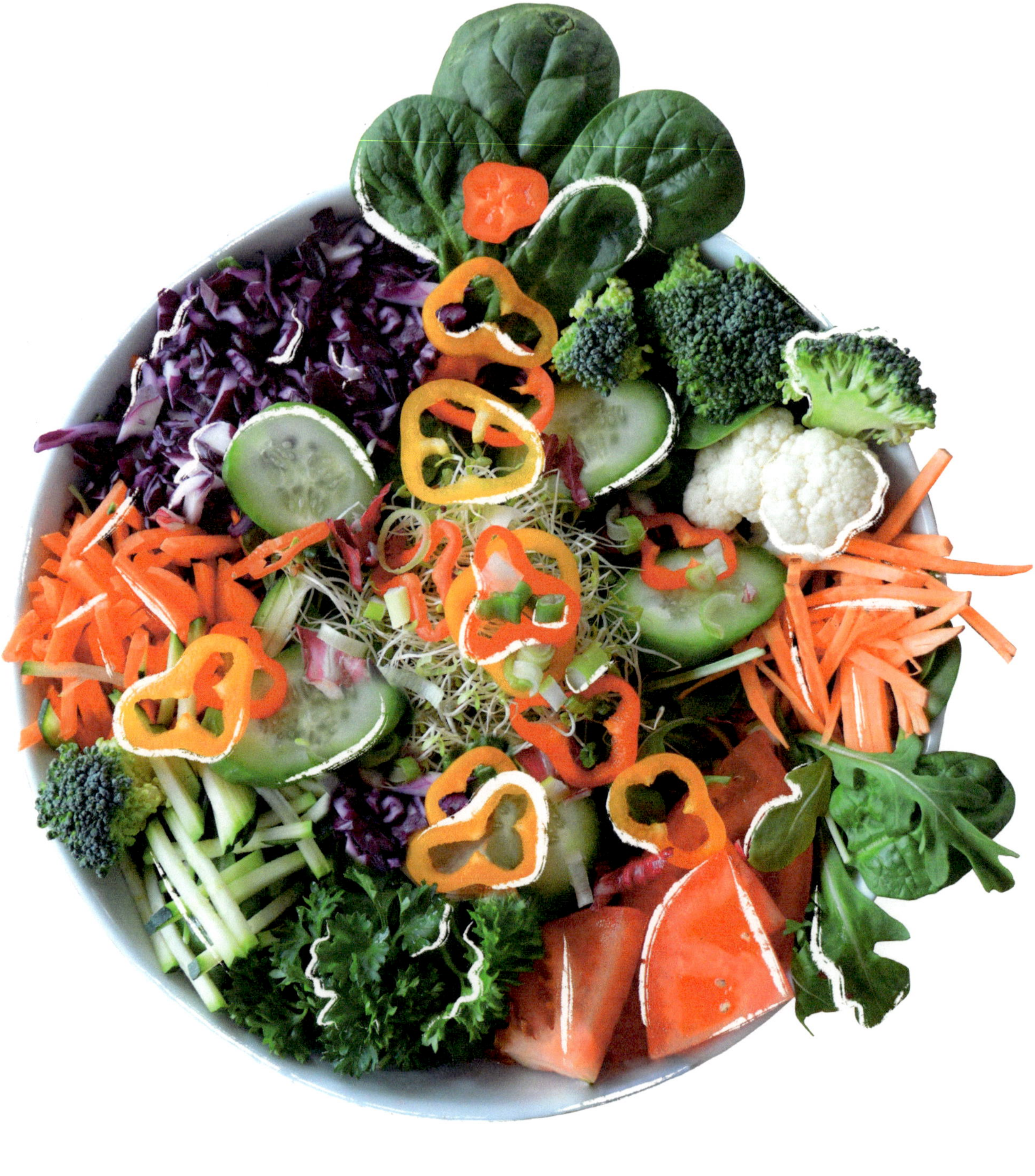

WHAT IS HEALTH?

HEALTH IS HOLISTIC. For instance, nutrition affects all of our body systems. Extra weight causes inflammation in your gut, and that poor gut health can lead to disease. And, there is a direct relationship between one's spinal health and the weight it carries. Extra weight affects the discs—causing herniations, protrusions, and arthritis. So, since we operate in a "non-ideal" world that is in a constant health crisis of obesity and the normalization of overeating, I am here to help.

This book is loaded with goodies: Ideal Advice and Ideal Actions, information, notes, recipes, and my own experience attaining my range of Ideal Weights. I actually created and designed this content with everyone in mind. . .but especially for those who are postmenopausal.

First, let's learn terms important to this book.

RELEVANT HEALTH TERMS

HEALTH comes from the Old English word "hale," meaning wholeness, being whole, sound, or well. The definition has evolved over the years; today the World Health Organization states that health "is a state of complete physical, mental and social well-being; not just the absence of disease." Simply put, health is an all-encompassing journey—not a destination.

IDEAL is defined as "satisfying one's conception of most suitable" and I believe your body—when following good health recommendations—can guide you to find and commit to a healthy weight. It is also defined as "perfection," but we have a more generous definition. Here are a few terms to know that involve good health.

POSITIVE HEALTH is a concept established in the 5th century by the Hippocratic physicians who were very interested in preventative measures for staying healthy. They also believed that positive health involves many aspects, including exercising, genetics, age, and environment. Deficiencies in any of these could contribute to one falling ill.

TWO "TYPES" OF FOOD is a way of looking at the "substances" we consume, as coined by Joshua Rosenthal.

PRIMARY FOOD is the kind of "food" that does not come on a plate. It consists of more complex elements, such as love, an exciting project, spirituality or high self-esteem. Imbalance of any of these can bring harm to ourselves, similar to binging and eating processed foods.

SECONDARY FOOD is the physical form of food that we consume. The healthier you eat, the fewer cravings you will have for processed foods. Discover which primary foods are missing and how to make room for joy and satisfaction into your life. Identifying imbalances will help you understand ways to spend more time and energy to create primary food balance, which will lead to positive secondary food choices.

BIO-INDIVIDUALITY is the idea that all beings are unique and individual. Ancestry, metabolic type, blood type, stress, constitution, environment, allergies, body composition, dietary habits, and illness over time are elements that make up our bio-individuality.

CLEAN EATING is exactly like it sounds, so do your best to avoid foods contaminated with pesticides via processing. According to the Mayo Clinic, "The fundamentals of eating clean encourage you to consume more whole foods such as fruits, vegetables, lean proteins, whole grains and healthy fats—and limit highly processed snack foods, sweets and other packaged foods."

SATIATION CUES can be defined by "the quality or state of being fed or gratified to or beyond capacity." Satiety is a peaceful fullness feeling. This book will show you how to tune into your natural cues and listen to your body.

Now, let's define a few HEALTH ISSUES.

CRAVINGS indicate consuming something that may or may not be good for us. It is an intense desire to consume a specific food, and is different from normal hunger; generally it feels uncontrollable. Areas of the brain that are responsible for memory and sensing pleasure are partially to blame for keeping those food cravings coming. According to the Monell Chemical Senses Center's research, the regions of the brain called the insula, the hippocampus, and caudate appear to be activated during food-craving episodes. Indeed, it is the same areas of the brain that are triggered in addiction.

GMO'S are genetically modified organisms. It is any organism (fruits, vegetables, meats, grains) or microorganism whose genetic material has been altered by means of genetic engineering. Generally, organic food cannot be a GMO—besides, your body instinctively knows how to process natural foods.

OVEREATING is taking in too much food. Food is fuel for your body. Do you ever pump gas into your car and when the tank is full, you just let it overflow? The same metaphor can be used with your body and overeating. Just as you refill your tank when it is empty, you should only eat when you are hungry. . .do not overfill!

PROCESSED FOODS are natural food that has been cooked, canned, frozen, packaged or changed in nutritional composition with fortifying, preserving, or preparing in different ways. Replace processed foods with natural whole foods. This will decrease cravings and allow you to refill when you are hungry. The healthier you eat, the less your body desires and commands—and that is how you control and maintain your weight.

TOXINS are defined by Merriam-Webster as "a poisonous substance that is a specific product of the metabolic activities of a living organism and is usually very unstable, notably toxic when

> ***NOTE:*** *A plethora of literature exists regarding nutritional theories. Ultimately, nutritional paths will vary and each person must find out what works for them on a bio-individual level.*

introduced into the tissues, and are typically capable of inducing inflammation or rejection." Essentially, toxins put pressure on the body's systems.

THE CHINA STUDY

THIS WELL-REGARDED STUDY WAS CONDUCTED by Thomas Campbell and T. Colin Campbell, reported in their book, *The China Study: The Most Comprehensive Study of Nutrition Ever Conducted and the Startling Implications for Diet, Weight Loss, and Long-term Health*. It explores the connection between animal products (including dairy) and chronic illnesses, putting forth the conclusion that Clean Eating as a predominantly whole-food, plant-based diet (when done while reducing processed foods) can diminish or even reverse some diseases.

FACTS FROM THE CHINA STUDY

- Two-thirds of Americans are overweight.
- One-third of children in the United States are overweight or at risk of becoming overweight.
- More than 15 million Americans have diabetes.
- More than 100 million Americans have high cholesterol.
- 3 trillion dollars is spent annually on healthcare.

All of these facts are alarming, but many of the issues are preventable with an overall healthy lifestyle.

Let's find out how!

IDEAL ACTION

Write down your own personal definitions of health. Think about why: *Why do we choose not to be healthy?* Dive into the "why" behind our poor decisions. By doing so, you will learn how to understand what healthy foods ultimately serve your body best.

Then, make a commitment and set realistic goals that motivate and excite you. Your goals should be challenging but not impossible. . .each goal needs a deadline to force you to stay focused. Deadlines are your friend!

MY STORY

MENOPAUSE CHANGED MY LIFE! My experience post menopause was positive. I learned how to truly treat myself well, lose weight naturally, and help others. I faced the challenges it presented, and not all of them with grace. Yet it taught me to destigmatize menopause and aging, as well as face scrutiny that comes with menopause and fat-shaming attacks against the female body.

MENOPAUSE IMPACTED MY REGULAR eating habits. In my early adulthood, I was able to consume most foods without suffering consequences. I had been eating processed food with added sugar unaware of the negative effects it had on my mind and body. At that time, however, I was able to cut calories and exercise to eliminate the excess weight.

Conversely, postmenopausal life is different. I have always wanted to look my best, and not being able to look and feel great after menopause drove me crazy. I went on yo-yo diets, and increased my exercise routine. . .to no avail. Out of desperation, I underwent surgical procedures including a tummy tuck. However, this was only a short-term fix, and I had to change my habits to avoid another surgical procedure.

ONE MIRACULOUS DAY, after suffering for only temporary changes, I realized I could change my life dramatically by shifting habits. And, I learned about the benefits of plant-based foods, which promoted permanence. This approach contradicted all of my previous dietary habits growing up. Once I switched over to the plant-based foods, I began to reach my ideal weight, which restored my confidence. Most of the people I know grew up eating rice and meat-based meals regularly—including me! During cultural holidays, family traditions, and religious observances at least one type of animal product is on most household tables. Throughout history, being able to feed livestock to your family was a sign of wealth and prosperity. Once I changed, my weight loss journey jump-started, and I discovered a new happiness.

THROUGH MY OWN HEALTH JOURNEY, I am able to support my patients. And, through watching their health improve, I am able to gather data that confirms my own experience, nutrition science, and my training.

Declining estrogen levels negatively impact your metabolism, potentially leading to weight gain. Shifting cholesterol levels can be difficult, and many women experience symptoms like hot flashes and difficulty sleeping during these changes. Fortunately, making changes in your diet may ease post menopause.

According to Healthline, "In a one-year intervention study, in over 17,000 menopausal women, those eating more vegetables, fruits, fiber, and soy experienced a 19% reduction in hot flashes compared to the control group." A healthier diet was found to create this reduction, as well as aiding in weight loss.

Weight gain and poor diet add to hot flashes. Therefore, you can decrease symptoms by proper food consumption and exercise. It begins with your mindset, then continues with the foods you bring into your kitchen, whether those foods are grocery-store bought or garden grown.

First believe—then achieve—*your* ideal weight!

THE BODY IS A MACHINE! But, as the body gets older, these miraculous machines need help. To eat well is to supply sustenance for a "body in transition." And, the fewer pounds you gain during menopause, the less problems will arise.

I became empowered once I knew I could improve my aging health. I knew that there was a mental aspect of giving up, simply *because it is menopause*. I realized that giving into it is a cop-out. I have been on the roller coaster, but now I am able to maintain my weight via food and exercise. Based on my own experiences and my patients' improvements, you can avoid gaining weight and instead achieve your own ideal weight.

SO, THE "PROOF IS IN THE PUDDING" (non-dairy, of course)!

DID YOU KNOW?

These foods create plant-based estrogen in the body: flax seeds, soybeans, chickpeas, peanuts, grapes, berries, plums, green, and black tea.

They contain natural phytoestrogens, thereby decreasing some uncomfortable outcomes of post menopause.

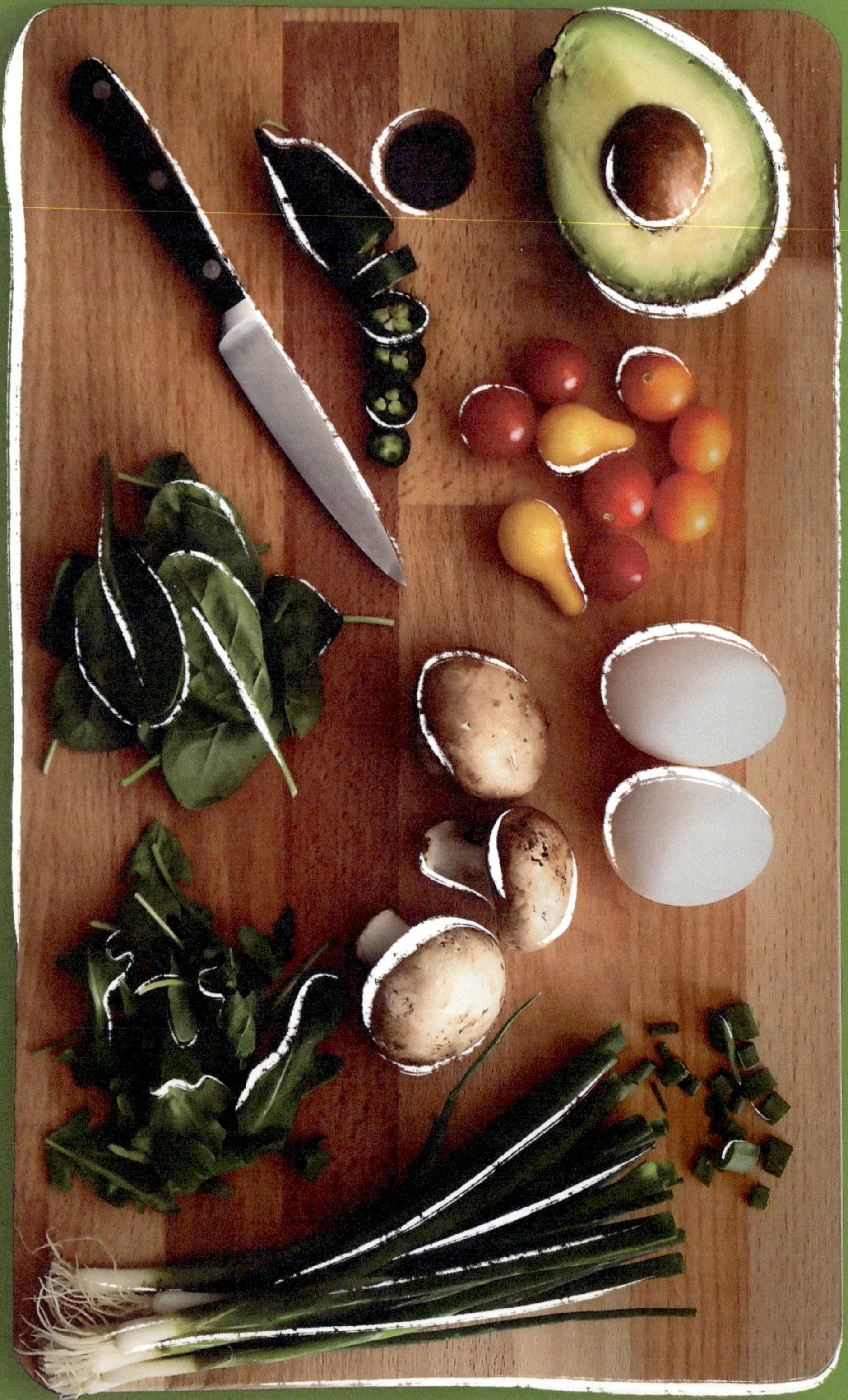

“LET FOOD BE THY MEDICINE AND MEDICINE BE THY FOOD.” -HIPPOCRATES

KNOW YOUR FOOD

MY COACHING AND WELLNESS techniques provide the groundwork and foundation needed to suit your specific needs. Additionally, I find that encouragement is an important aspect of a maintaining a healthy lifestyle. Finally, I recommend avoiding daily weigh-ins as it is initially discouraging and will deviate your focus from replacing unhealthy foods.

A HEALTHY LIFESTYLE HABIT will change your taste buds, increase your palate sensitivity, which ultimately promotes mindful food choices and consumption.

CLEAN EATING: HOW TO START

FIRST AND FOREMOST, CLEAN EATING takes practice and patience. Eating various colors of fruits and specific vegetables ensure that you are consuming the proper intake of vitamins and nutrients.

- **RED FRUITS** and vegetables support your heart and brain function.
- **ORANGE FRUITS** and veggies are full of beta carotene and vitamin C, which are great for eye health and immunity.
- **YELLOW FRUITS** and vegetables help improve circulation.
- **DEEP GREEN FRUITS** and vegetables purify the blood, strengthen the immune system, nourish the nervous system, and ward off depression and anxiety.
- **BLUE AND PURPLE** foods are rich in antioxidants and can prevent early signs of aging and heart disease.
- **WHITE FRUITS** and vegetables reduce blood pressure and LDL cholesterol.

Also, it is important to choose local, seasonal, or organic produce as often as possible.

- Keep fresh herbs, garlic, onions, and ginger in your refrigerator year round. These are known for their antiviral and antibacterial properties and often are used as natural antibiotics and they can enhance the food flavor.
- Load up on sweet vegetables, as they reduce sweet cravings. Say goodbye to cookies, cakes and ice cream! Sweeter cooked vegetables such as delicata squash, butternut squash, carrots, sweet potatoes, and onions can crowd out the junk food with real nourishment.
- Be sure to check the dates when buying fresh animal products. Look for the terms "organic," "free-range" or "cage-free," and "certified humane" on labels.

A CLEAN EATING FOUNDATION

PLANT-BASED PROTEIN

TOFU is soybean curd, it is a popular vegan meat substitute, for it even takes on the flavor of any seasoning you add to it.

SEITAN is a vegan protein made of wheat gluten. If you are allergic to soy but not to wheat, it may be a good protein for you.

TEMPEH is made of whole soybeans fermented into a block. It has a toasted, nutty flavor that is perfect for grilling or stir frying.

BEANS AND LEGUMES are some of the most cost effective protein sources available. Not only are they a great source of protein, they are also a great source of fiber, magnesium, and iron.

SEEDS: Chia seeds have 5.1 grams of protein per ounce, flaxseed oil has 7.3 grams per 1 tablespoon serving, and walnuts contain 2.6 grams per ounce. These are also some of the best plant sources of omega-3 fatty acids—excellent for your heart and brain health.

ANIMAL PROTEINS

SALMON, COD, SARDINES, AND MACKEREL are the better sources of fish for consumption; smaller fish tend to swim closer to the surface of water and carry less mercury.

When buying whole fish, take a good look at the eyes and gills; the eyes should be clear, not glazed over, and the gills should be red. Fish should also have tight skin and a clean smell. Fish fillet and steaks should be bright and clean in color—not murky. Always ask when the fish came in, and if it has been sitting on display for more than a day you might want to consider other options.

EGGS are a complete protein, they provide all essential amino acids the body needs. They are a great source of protein, especially when added to a meal of grains and vegetables. Look for "certified organic," "free-range," "certified humane," and "Grade A pastured" on the package.

DAIRY can be controversial. Many argue that it can lead to digestive issues, allergies, or mucus, while others enjoy dairy symptom free. Experiment with dairy and see how it affects you. Choose high-quality products labeled "pasture-raised," "free-range," "organic," or "grass-fed."

If dairy does not work for you, other options are soy (non-GMO), rice, oat, coconut, hemp, and a number of nut milks including almond and hazelnut. When choosing non-dairy milk, purchase as unsweetened as possible and pick labels with the fewest number of ingredients.

GHEE is used like butter, it adds a delicious nutty flavor to vegetables and can be added to grains after they have been cooked. Ghee also can help balance excess stomach acids.

WHOLE GRAINS

WHEAT GRAINS include bulgur, cracked wheat, spelt, and wheat berries. However, products that claim that they are "whole grain" should list a pure whole grain first, not a name like "enriched wheat" or "enriched flour."

WHEAT-FREE AND GLUTEN-FREE grains include amaranth, buckwheat, millet, rice, quinoa. Oats are inherently gluten free but look for "certified gluten-free."

OILS

OILS are basically fats that are needed for everything from brain function to vitamin absorption. However, you CAN get great healthy fats from oils, nuts, seeds, coconuts, and avocados. In choosing oils, follow this advice.

- Avoid oils that are hydrogenated or bleached.
- Look for brands that are cold-pressed and unrefined.
- Olive oil is great for salads and grains.
- Sesame oil has a nutty flavor.
- Coconut oil has a smooth coconut taste.
- Almond oil, avocado oil, hazelnut oil, and high-oleic sunflower oil are also options.

CONDIMENTS

HEALTHY SUGGESTIONS INCLUDE: Gluten-free soy sauce like tamari, apple cider vinegar, balsamic vinegar, hot pepper, sesame oil, cayenne pepper, hot sauce, tahini, nut butters, and nutritional yeast (which has a cheesy flavor that is loaded with protein and B vitamins).

HERBS AND SPICES

HERBS AND SPICES ARE FULL OF MEDICINE and flavor! Basil, oregano, thyme, and bay leaves are great on whole grain bread with garlic and olive oil. They also complement meat. Coriander, cumin, ginger, cardamom, and nutmeg enhances the flavor of vegetables and makes them more digestible. They can also improve the digestion of dairy, fruits, and desserts.

STEVIA is a natural plant extract. It contains zero calories, is 200 times sweeter than sugar and will not raise blood glucose (blood sugar) level. Use in small amounts.

SALT should also be used in small amounts. Choose either pink Himalayan or naturally harvested sea salt.

"Food is a gift and should be treated reverentially—romanced and ritualized and seasoned with memory." -Chris Bohjalian

CURB CRAVINGS

"BUT, WHAT ABOUT MY CRAVINGS?" is a common question I receive. People either feel attached to their comfort foods or believe that it is impossible to give up the habit. Cravings are an addiction as well!

Below is a chart of the possible causes behind your cravings and suggestions for other healthier food replacements.

DEFINING A CRAVING

MERRIAM-WEBSTER'S DEFINITION OF THE TERM "craving" is an intense, urgent, or abnormal desire or longing. Here, it applies to unhealthier food choices or amount of consumption.

OUR BODY IS A BIO-COMPUTER. However, like other computers, glitches exist in the form of unhealthy cravings. Luckily, eating healthy can include a rewarding INDULGE MEAL. Indulge meals can be executed in various ways, but one example would be to create a healthier version of your craving. So long as you are conscious of your craving, it is possible to enjoy the craving without feeling guilty!

ASK YOURSELF: *AM I ACTUALLY HUNGRY* or is there another explanation (or underlying reason) for overeating?

One light meal and a few healthy snacks throughout the day will suffice if executed properly. You can avoid that uncomfortable "stuffed" feeling from overfilling on non-nutritious foods.

THERE IS NO SECRET TO WEIGHT LOSS. A well-fed and nutrient-filled body will reduce unhealthy cravings, since it allows the body to feel satiated fast. The answers to your problems do not have to be found in the "comfort" foods of your pantry or local takeout.

CRAVINGS & DEFICIENCIES CHART

CRAVING:	POSSIBLE MISSING NUTRIENT:	RECOMMENDED REPLACEMENT:
chocolate	magnesium	raw nuts, seeds
sugar	chromium, carbon, tryptophan, phosphorous	broccoli, beans, kale, cranberries, raisins, sweet potatoes, spinach
bread	nitrogen	nuts, beans
fatty foods	calcium	broccoli, mustard greens, kale, sesame
ice	iron	seaweed, greens
charred foods	carbon	fresh fruit

IDEAL ADVICE

Hunger is tricky. Cravings are confused signals that disturb your hunger and satiety. They can mask your true urge to eat well and eat less. Here are tips to help you conquer cravings!

- Protein is your friend! Consume protein-rich, plant-based foods and snacks as they will provide an energy-filled and power-sourced body all day.
- Shake it 'til you make it. High-plant protein shakes will also fill you and enable better eating choices.
- Recognize the craving—then master it by using mindfulness and digestion science.
- Drink a glass of water or hot tea. When feeling hungry, you might actually be thirsty!
- Exercise. Any movement counts! The more you move, the more your metabolism will support your weight goal.
- Be your own Portion Patrol. Enable your satiation cues to guide you toward a fulfilling portion and away from overeating.
- Decrease stress through meditation. Meditation can train the muscle of the brain how to focus, switch tracks of thinking, and therefore make better decisions.
- Sleep is medicine!
- Spend time with good friends; this can help take up time and increase mood, so you will be less likely to indulge in overeating or emotional eating.
- Drink sugarless and dairy-free coffee with a milk-substitute, such as almond milk.
- Eat more dark chocolate. Dark chocolate stimulates taste receptors and circulates ghrelin, which regulates hunger. The more dark and bitter the chocolate is, the better.

IDEAL ACTION

Keep a food journal throughout your weight loss journey. Do at least 5 of the above-mentioned recommendations for a week. Start to notice the difference. Trust your gut about what feels the best and what foods provide the best energy. As you track your eating, your food awareness will increase.

ATTACK FOOD ADDICTION

WHAT IS FOOD ADDICTION?

IN ORDER TO UNDERSTAND more about cravings and compulsive binge eating, let's turn to the Yale Food Addiction Study. This groundbreaking work took the same criteria for determining substance abuse and drug addiction and applied it to the way we consume food.

THE YALE FOOD ADDICTION QUESTIONNAIRE

- Do you consume foods even if you are not hungry because of cravings?
- Do you worry about cutting down on certain foods?
- Do you feel sluggish or fatigued from overeating?
- Do you have health or social problems (affecting school or work) because of food issues and yet keep eating the way you do?
- Do you spend time dealing with negative feelings from overeating certain foods?
- Do you have withdrawal symptoms such as agitation and anxiety when you cut down on certain foods?
- Does your behavior around food and eating cause you significant distress?
- Do food issues decrease your availability to function effectively?
- Do you need more and more of the foods you crave to experience pleasure or reduce negative emotions?

Did you answer "yes" to any of the questions? If so, you are not alone! This leads us to another question: What is the difference between a drug addict and a food addict? Not much, actually, in terms of brain activation. Studies have shown that sugar and junk foods flood the reward system in the brain with dopamine, "the feel-good" chemical we make (and often seek out), stimulating the same areas lit up by using drugs such as cocaine. If any of this doesn't sound ideal. . .well, it isn't.

You deserve better flow and control of your life around food! So, keep reading, I can help!

NOTE: *It is best to buy foods with fewer total ingredients and names that are easier to understand. Rethink your decision when you notice multiple ingredients with complex names that are difficult to pronounce.*

DID YOU KNOW?

Binge eating is a common symptom of food addiction. It is caused by tolerance, making the brain require a larger amount than before in order to reach the same effect.

WHAT ARE THE MOST ADDICTIVE FOODS?

THESE FOODS ARE TYPICALLY TASTY (enjoyable at first), but can create havoc on our system. Here is a list—avoid as many as you can.

CASEIN: dairy-containing foods are addictive. Cheese is the culprit here, as are heavy fats like ice cream.

GLUTEN is in so many carbohydrates, such as breads, cakes, pastries. While we associate it most with wheat, it is in many other grains like oats (due to contamination in the processing). Look for a GF stamp on packaging.

SUGAR affects the brain by increasing the release of dopamine, which is a neurotransmitter that creates a pleasurable feeling. An increased release of this same neurotransmitter is seen in those who use heroin, cocaine, and opioids. Imaging studies have also compared drug-addicted brains and sugar-addicted brains. . . and the end result is that they look the same. Furthermore, research on sugar and sugar substitutes show that they are four times more addictive than cocaine.

HIGH FRUCTOSE CORN SYRUP

- Twice as sweet and addictive as sucrose (table sugar).
- Equally capable of causing liver damage as alcohol.

SWEETENERS

Beware! Artificial sweeteners falsely stimulate your taste receptors so that the brain constantly craves sugar.

- These raise blood sugar and can cause digestive problems, especially when artificial or lab-created.
- Common artificial sweeteners to avoid:
  - aspartame acesulfame potassium (Equal)
  - sucralose (Splenda)
  - saccharin (Sweet n' Low)
  - dextrose
  - maltodextrin
  - maltitol (sugar alcohol)
  - sorbitol (sugar alcohol)

IDEAL ACTION

In your journal, write down the 5 most addicting foods you *will* overcome.

Build your mindfulness around what you are consuming.

When reaching for food to eat, stop, breathe, and slow down.

Drink water or tea.

Ask yourself: *Do I really need this, or am I just being tricked because I am stressed or just overly tired?*

Create an affirmation: *I now overcome this craving*. Repeat out loud.

WEIGHT & WELLNESS

IN THE UNITED STATES ALONE, an estimated two-thirds of the population is considered overweight or obese, putting their health at risk. Because this issue is spreading throughout the globe, it is important to find ways to help reduce its prevalence and encourage individuals to develop healthy habits. I am here to help!

Originally, I considered changing my eating habits when I began to struggle with my weight and recurrent hemorrhoids. I felt sadness and a decline in self-confidence. When medications would only temporarily treat my problems, I became a vegan that eats eggs—called ovo-vegan— to see if this would help. Within the first week of the new lifestyle change, my hemorrhoid was completely gone! Moreover, my cravings decreased significantly.

Because of my positive results, I decided to continue Clean Eating and have since lost 26 pounds. I feel lighter and less bloated and my mind is more clear. And, a recent blood test also revealed that I am on the right health path. Yes, you too can do this!

WHAT IS AN IDEAL WEIGHT?

IDEAL WEIGHT IS ANY WEIGHT at which one feels the healthiest (while maintaining the state safely and sustainably). Now, since each body is different and ever-changing, you may reach one ideal weight and then another! I created Ideal Weights because I know there can be a range: you can reach a goal, sustain it, and even improve upon it! There are two ways to determine a general number. Please connect with whichever method works for you. No matter what, be gentle on yourself. You may not be at your desired weight yet, but you can still act ideally by being patient with your goals.

> ***NOTE:*** *If you want to use animal products, I recommend that you purchase organic, grass-fed, hormone-free, and antibiotic-free products. You do not need to eat animal protein for every meal. For instance, there are enough proteins in legumes to satisfy your intake. I am not suggesting everyone become vegetarians or vegans, however, I have researched that in the United States the obesity epidemic and other diseases have been linked to frequent consumption of animal products.*

1. THE FIRST WAY IS A TECHNICAL EQUATION. In general, being within 10% of this number is considered acceptable in order to allow for different body types.

WOMEN: Start with 100 pounds + 5 pounds each inch you are above 5 feet and - 5 pounds for each inch below 5 feet.

Men: Start with 106 pounds + 6 pounds for each inch you are above 5 feet and - 6 pounds for each inch below 5 feet.

2. THE SECOND WAY IS INTUITIVE. Focusing strictly on body weight can create a stressful relationship with food, physical activity, and overall lifestyle. Do not become obsessed with the number on the scale! Follow your intuition. This allows people to dictate the path of their health journey versus relying on standardized numbers set forth by others. Bodyweight is only a small portion of the wellness puzzle.

CRASH EATING VS. JUST EATING WELL

OBESITY OCCURS WHEN A PERSON CONSUMES more calories from eating than they burn. Counting calories in weight loss can be done in short periods of time, but learning to eliminate the unhealthy, processed foods—and instead turn your focus on eating nutrient-dense foods—will help you balance your weight.

IDEAL ADVICE

Simply start by making 1-3 small changes in your diet. Try to refrain from drinking soda and consuming dairy and desserts for two weeks. Try not eating after 6:00-7:00 pm.

You can do it! Remember that you deserve to feel better. After the two weeks, your *palate sensitivity* will increase. As a result, your cravings for soda, dairy, and dessert will change because they will no longer taste as satisfying.

Discover the emotional component behind overeating. Overeating happens for many, even for me when stress is overwhelming.

I encourage you to make a decision to become aware of what stimulates your overeating by re-evaluating parts of your life: relationships, career, love, personal finances, mindset, and time management.

Once you uncover the underlying cause of your overeating and therefore empower yourself, reaching your goals will not be an issue.

EASY TIPS FOR WEIGHT LOSS

- Focus on a reliable change instead of instant results; be kind and patient with yourself.
- Limit involvement with fad diets—your body knows best when given the chance!
- Remember that food deprivation as seen in fad diets typically backfires.
- Keep a food journal to create more mindful awareness.
- Know your options, choose wisely. Educate yourself! Listen to your body.
- Keep your meals small and frequent.
- Chew your food slowly. Try counting the bites one by one.
- Eat when you are hungry; learn when you are truly hungry.
- Cook food at home, this will eliminate indulging in comfort foods, as well as lowering consumption of processed foods and additives.
- Drink 8 cups of fluids (mostly water).
- Sip seltzer or club soda in lieu of regular soda to reduce sugar and caloric intake.
- Switch from whole milk to almond milk—nut milks contain protein!
- Try a plant-based protein powder for decreased cravings.
- Choose 100% fresh fruit juice; However, drink no more than 4 ounces 2-3 times a week.
- Refrain from fancy, sugary latte drinks.
- No more than 1 glass of wine/beer/cocktail a day to avoid system stress and calories.
- Eat a variety of legumes. Legumes add protein without major calories.
- Get enough sleep. Most adults need 7-9 hours of sleep per night. Sleeping allows the body to

recuperate. Therefore, you will have fewer cravings and be able to make better decisions.

- Exercise your body—any movement counts! This results in looser joints, more energy and less stagnancy, leading to better decisions.

FOODS THAT PROMOTE WEIGHT LOSS:

- almonds
- blackberries
- cayenne pepper
- coconut meat
- cucumbers
- peaches
- sauerkraut
- fermented foods
- apple cider vinegar
- bok choy
- chia seeds
- coconut oil
- hemp seeds
- tart cherries
- brussels sprouts
- chickpeas
- lemons
- nectarines
- pumpkin seeds

FOODS THAT PROMOTE SATIETY:

- brazil nuts
- chickpeas
- pickles
- pine nuts
- boiled potatoes
- eggs
- oatmeal
- soups

IDEAL ACTION

Choose 10 of these foods from the Foods That Promote Weight Loss and Foods That Promote Satiety lists. To eat plant-based foods is to eat guilt-free.

Bon appétit!

SNACKING SYSTEM

SNACKING—WE ALL ENJOY IT. In fact, a snack can be fun *and* nutritious too!

PORTION CONTROL IS ALWAYS IMPORTANT to remember, so as not to strain the digestive system. The portions mentioned here—if followed properly—will help with weight loss.

SNACKING SUGGESTIONS

- Try two tablespoons of natural almond butter with apple slices, celery sticks, or rice cakes.
- Eat sliced carrots, snap peas, cucumber with 2 tablespoons of hummus.
- Enjoy ¼ cup of either raw or soaked almonds or walnuts. I recommend soaking these overnight, rinsing the next morning, and then eating a fistful every day. Grab them for on-the-go eating!
- Have ¼ cup of pistachios, macadamia nuts, pumpkin or sunflower seeds.
- Make homemade zucchini or kale chips that have been battered in avocado oil.
- Eat black or green olives.
- Enjoy a ½ cup of quinoa. Quinoa is full of protein and is very satisfying.
- Eat a ½ cup of guacamole and sliced vegetables.
- Crunch 1-2 dill pickles. Pickles will set your taste receptors. Anything fermented helps digestion!

AND DON'T FORGET DELICIOUS FRUITS that fill you up while not adding tons of calories.

LOW-CALORIE FRUITS:

- watermelon
- pear
- apple
- blueberries
- pineapple
- strawberries
- avocado
- cantaloupe
- avocados
- honeydew
- peaches

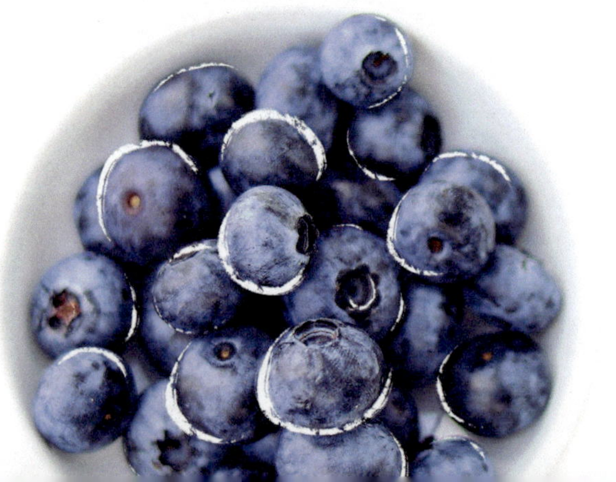

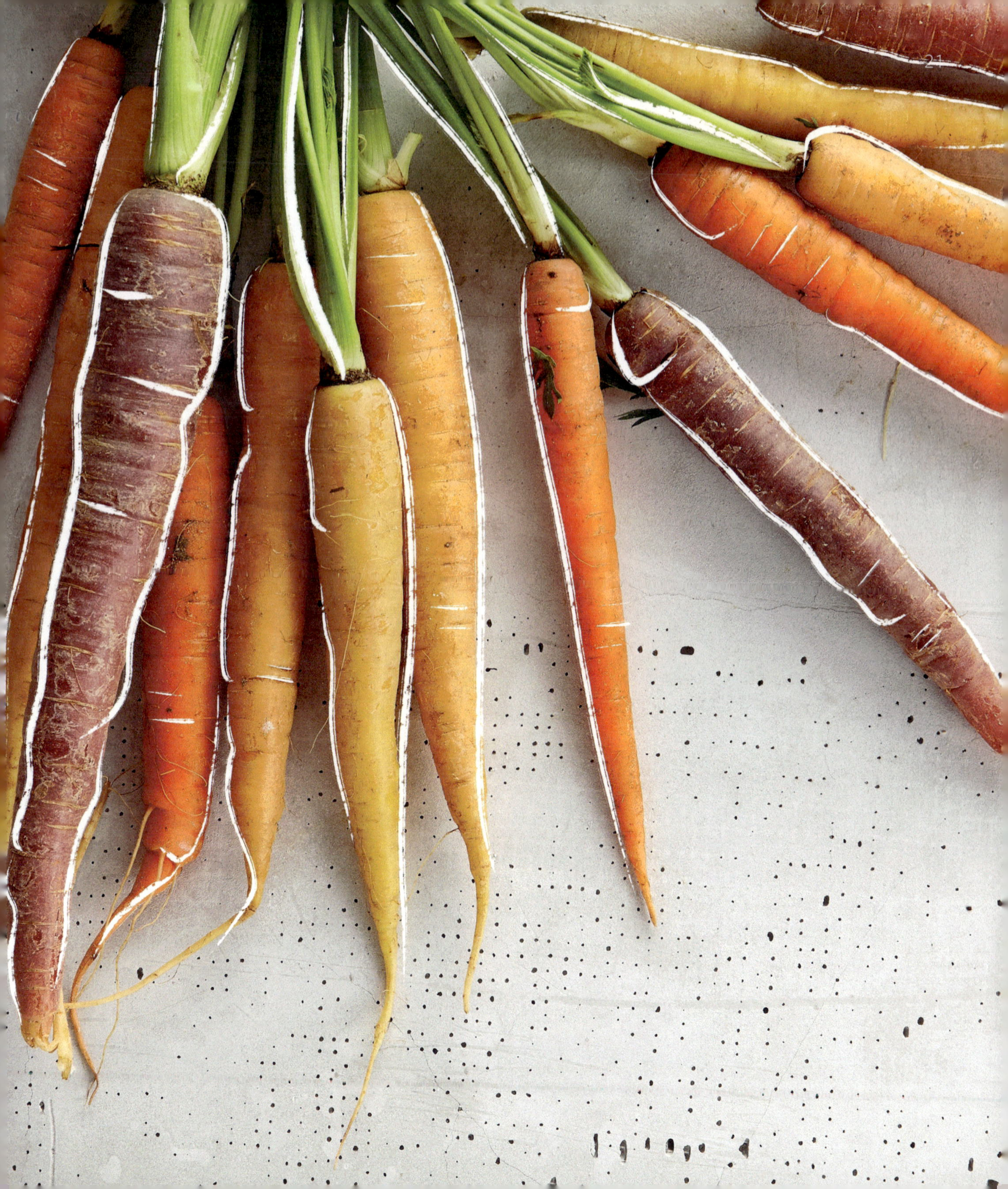

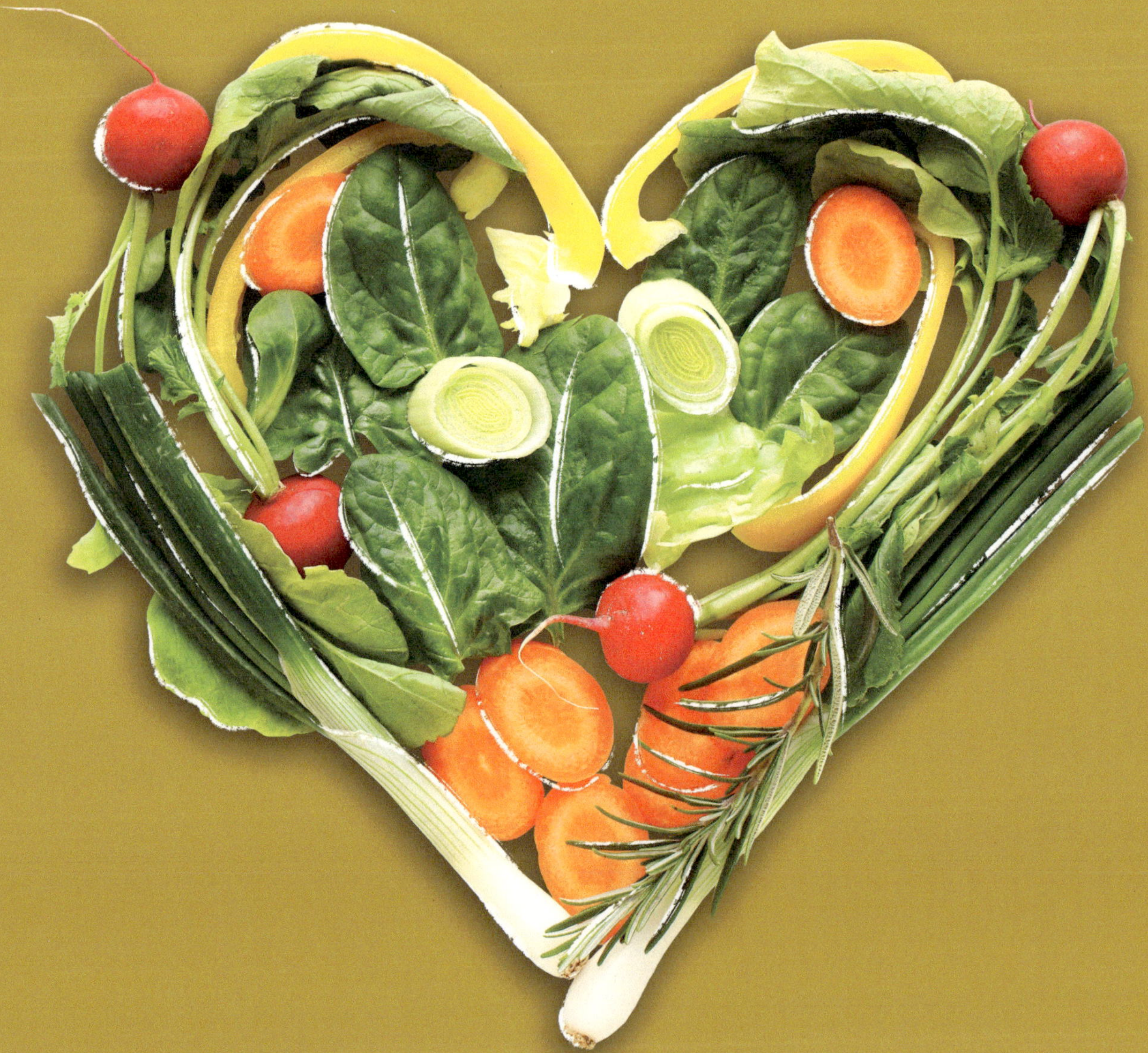

"LOVE YOUR BODY BECAUSE YOU ONLY HAVE ONE."

-ANONYMOUS

KNOW YOUR BODY

NOW THAT YOU ARE MORE WELL-INFORMED to make better food choices, you can begin your journey towards a healthier lifestyle. An important factor of weight loss involves absorbing information about your body.

ALL OF YOUR BODY AND ITS SYSTEMS are affected by food choices and nutrition. I encourage you to learn more about these incredible systems working so hard for you. The more you understand, the more you can attain health alongside peak performance.

BODY SYSTEMS

- Skeletal
- Muscular
- Gastrointestinal
- Respiratory
- Urinary
- Circulatory
- Lymphatic
- Reproductive
- Endocrine
- Nervous system
- Integumentary

Knowledge is power on this health journey! Read on to learn more about the intricacies of your body and its optimal function.

BMR & BMI

GOOD NEWS: YOU CAN UNDERSTAND your body by calculating metabolism and measuring your body mass. The more you know, the more you can change! Start by calculating your BMR and BMI.

CALCULATE YOUR BASAL METABOLIC RATE (BMR)

BMR IS THE NUMBER OF CALORIES needed at rest to maintain your current weight and for your body to accomplish its most basic functions to sustain life (i.e. breathing, circulation, nutrient processing, and cell production). One great way to avoid fad diet products and to lose weight on your own in a sustainable way is to calculate your BMR and know your status. Then, by eating 500-1000 fewer calories a day, you can lose 1-2 pounds a week. Empower yourself with information!

HARRIS-BENEDICT FORMULA FOR CALCULATING BMR

Women
655 + (9.6 x weight in kilograms)+(1.85 x height in centimeters) - (4.7 x age in years).

Men
66 + (13.7 x weight in kilograms) +(5 x height in centimeters) - (6.8 x age in years).

Now, once you know that, you can discover how many calories you need daily.

> ***NOTE:*** *The number of calories a person needs depends on many factors, such as: age, height, body composition, weight history, gender, overall state of health, and general levels of activity.*

If you are:

Sedentary: Minimal (or no exercise), multiply your BMR by 1.2.

Lightly active: Exercise lightly (3 days a week), multiply your BMR by 1.375.

Moderate active: Exercise (3-5 times a week), multiply your BMR by 1.55.

Very active: Hard exercise (6-7 times a week), multiply your BMR by 1.725.

Extra active: Very hard exercise (6-7 days a week), or have a physical job, multiply your BMR by 1.9.

STANDARD FOR CALORIC INTAKE

Women: (18 years +) = 1800 - 2400 calories (does not apply to pregnant and breastfeeding women).

Men: (18 years +) = 2400 - 3200 calories.

CALCULATE YOUR BODY MASS INDEX (BMI)

YOUR BMI WHICH IS THE AMOUNT OF FAT on one's body. This is based on an adult's weight and height The higher the BMI, the greater the risk of developing diabetes, high blood pressure, heart disease, and early death. To calculate it take your weight in kilograms and divide it by your height in meters squared or BMI- kg/m2.

$$BMI = \frac{\text{weight (kg)}}{[\text{height}]\ \text{meters}^2}$$

Or you can calculate it using your weight in pounds times 703, divided by your height in inches squared.

$$BMI = \frac{(\text{weight in pounds}) \times (703)}{(\text{height in inches})^2}$$

You can also google BMI calculator online. Here below, you can see your "status" and work on that, empowering yourself with basic standards.

STANDARD CLASSIFICATION OF BMI

If you are:

Below 18-19 = underweight.
19-25 = healthy weight (low health risk).
25-30 = overweight (moderate health risk).
30-40 = obese (high health risk).
Over 40 = morbid obesity (very high health risk).

ESTIMATED DAILY PROTEIN NEEDED TO MAINTAIN CURRENT WEIGHT

For example, (sedentary) women need 46 grams of protein per day, while (sedentary) men require 56 grams of protein per day. You can also multiply 0.36 by your weight in pounds to achieve the amount of protein needed. If you have kidney disease or engage in minimal physical activity, the amount of need decreases.

SUGGESTED CALORIC INTAKE FOR WEIGHT LOSS

Women: Non-active = 1000 – 1200 calories.
Active = 1200 1500 calories.

Men: Non-active = 1200 – 1500 calories
Active = 1500 – 1800 calories.

Teenagers: 1200 – 1800 calories.

The above amounts will allow for 1-2 pounds of weight loss a week.

FASTING FRAMEWORK

INTERMITTENT FASTING IS A GREAT WAY to lose weight and gain health. The concept is to start your first meal between 11:00 am-12:00 pm and finish your last meal no later than 7:00 pm. This will provide you with a 16-hour fast between the last meal and the next meal the following day.

Studies show that even practicing this a few days a week benefits your health, as long as there is a 14-16 hour fast between the last meal of the day and the first meal on the next day.

A FEW YEARS AGO, I BEGAN FOCUSING on eating plant-based foods. . .and to my surprise, I lost 15 pounds in one month without feeling hungry or as if I was depriving myself. I used positive self-talk and coached myself to move forward with every decision. I really wanted to build on my achievements and positive feelings.

Now in addition to a plant-based diet, drinking water, and light exercise, I embrace Intermittent Fasting. Between the hours of 11:00 am-6:00 pm, I eat reasonably portioned plant-based foods, (which are highlighted throughout this book).

CHANGING MY EATING HABITS caused my body to adjust and crave healthier meals, as opposed to junk food. When I stopped eating in the evening until late the next morning, my body was given a chance to use fat for energy.

BENEFITS OF INTERMITTENT FASTING

THERE ARE MANY BENEFITS to reap from Intermittent Fasting, especially if you want to establish a lifestyle that promotes wellness. Daily fasting can stimulate important cellular repair processes as well as alter hormone levels that make your body—and all that it stores—more able to burn fat. Positive results from fasting include the following points.

- Insulin levels drop: Blood levels of insulin drop significantly, which facilitates fat burning.
- Human growth hormone revs up: This natural growth hormone makes fat-burning possible.
- Cellular repair occurs as waste is removed.

> ***NOTE:*** *You may consume liquids, such as coffee, preferably decaf and organic. I recommend using milk substitutes for your creamer (i.e. hemp milk, almond milk, coconut milk).Water and teas that are decaf and organic are healthy alternatives.*

- Overall health improves: Longevity and protection against disease increases.

BREAK-THE-FAST: BREAKFAST

IT IS VERY IMPORTANT TO BREAK YOUR FAST wisely, as the first meal sets up the tone for the rest of the day. This creates fewer cravings and helps maintain weight loss much easier.

EVEN THOUGH IT IS COMMON to wake up and immediately eat breakfast, a healthier alternative is to wait until noon to break your fast, allowing your body to tap into your visceral fat cells. Instead of eating right away, start your morning with 20 ounces of warm (or room temperature) water. Drink as much as 60 ounces throughout the morning. This is a great appetite suppressant and gives you a sensation of satiation!

Next, have a small cup of coffee (preferably organic) or hot tea (preferably decaffeinated and organic) with steamed almond milk and a small amount of cinnamon. Personally, I drink about 40-60 ounces of water along with a cup of organic coffee with almond milk throughout the morning.

Many find it difficult at first to wait until 11:00 am-12:00 pm to eat. If that is the case, gradually push back your breakfast by an hour every couple of days in order for your body to adjust to the change. Around 11:00 am, I have my first meal, which is typically one of the following: brown rice with black beans and avocado, a salad with 1-2 types of legumes, a cup of steamed vegetables with a cup of lentils, a salad with 1-2 eggs, a vegetable omelet, or tofu with sautéed vegetables.

Then, be sure to plan the last meal of the day to be no later than 6:00-7:00 pm. You may still have liquids such as water or hot tea after your dinner, but solid foods are not recommended within this particular method. Chewing wakes up the hunger center in your brain. Start practicing this and you will soon adjust to a healthier you!

QUICKSTART YOUR WEIGHT LOSS

- Avoid the following foods.
  - Processed foods and snacks. Go for nuts and your favorite fruits instead!
  - Carbohydrates (bread, potatoes, cereal, baked goods, etcetera).
  - High-sodium foods (deli meats, cereals, canned foods).
  - Heavy fats like bacon. These clog your system.
  - Items rich in sugar and fats (i.e. candy, fast food, soda).
  - Chewing gum or having mints.
  - Snacking between meals.

- Drink 1-2 glasses of water half an hour before each meal. Drink water whenever you feel hungry and before eating any solid foods. Water helps fill up the stomach and lessens hunger feelings.

- Begin an Intermittent Fasting practice at least a few days a week.

- Chew your food slowly; the more you chew, the less your body has to break down. Staying mindful and chewing really well in the mouth aids in digestion.

- Be mindful of what is on your plate; do not over serve with large portions.

- Use smaller plates; this will help with smaller portions.

- Use chopsticks; these can help one not load in mouthfuls and scarf down food.

- Sleep longer to digest better. Do not eat beforehand to give your digestive system a chance to rest.

- Sleep between 7-9 hours a day.

- Sleep in cold temperatures to burn more calories; this can also diminish hot flash feelings.
- Sit at a table to eat instead of in front of the television; this will create mindfulness.
- Add fat-burning foods (nuts, olive oil, hot peppers) and herbs (green tea, turmeric, basil, garlic) to your cooking.
- Add fiber to your foods, like dark green leafy vegetables and chia seeds.
- Add appetite suppressants like avocado, sweet potatoes (grilled or baked), apples, jicama, dark chocolate (that is dark or contains over 70% cocoa).
- Do not ever feel food deprived. Eat anytime you want (in your 8-10 hour window), but have smaller portions. Less is more!
- Diminish stress as best you can. Take up meditation and positive self talk.
- Add metabolic boosters, such as cinnamon and ginger, and herbs like cumin, rosemary, cayenne pepper, oregano, cardamom. Do not use more than 1-2 teaspoons of these herbs combined. If you are consuming these herbs in the form of supplements, use the recommended dosage. (Just because they are natural does not mean you should over-consume them).

SLEEP STRATEGIES

SLEEP. THE PLACE WE DREAM. Something we do every night. Indeed, it is a process we take for granted, or something we often give up in an effort to work and do more.

As David Rapoport, MD, (and director of the NYU Sleep Disorder program), states: "Sleep used to be kind of ignored, like parking our car in a garage and picking it up in the morning." But that is not the case anymore. Sleep, as it turns out, is more important than we thought. Sleep science continues to find out more about its relationship to health, and even sleep experts now help people get better sleep!

BENEFITS OF A SOLID NIGHT'S SLEEP

- Improved memory.
- Increased attention span.
- Expanded longevity.
- Added anti-aging effects.
- Support in maintaining a healthy weight.
- Decreased stress.
- Natural antidepressant.

THE RELATIONSHIP BETWEEN SLEEP & WEIGHT

STUDIES SHOW THAT FEWER THAN 7 hours of sleep significantly increases the risk of obesity.

RATES OF LOST SLEEP IN RELATION TO INCREASED WEIGHT

- 6 hours of sleep = 27% increase.
- 5 hours of sleep = 73% increase.
- Children (ages 6 -12):
  - Fewer than 10 hours of sleep a night may lead to 3.5 times greater incidence of obesity compared to 12 hours.
  - Sleep deprivation at 30 months of age can predict obesity by age 6.

RISKS ASSOCIATED WITH A LACK OF SLEEP *cited from Mark Hyman, MD*

WHEN WE LOSE SLEEP, especially the "good kind," our bodies are more prone to having a range of issues, such as the ones listed here.

- Increased inflammation.
- Increased amounts of cortisol—the stress hormone.
- Reduced leptin. This mimics starvation and hunger, creating cues that urge us to eat.
- Increased ghrelin—the hunger hormone.
- Activated reward systems that boost cravings and addiction behavior.

All of these increase the chances of gaining weight and becoming a diabetic, not to mention that lost sleep affects your mood!

IDEAL ADVICE

SLEEP HYGIENE

- Keep your bedroom well-ventilated and between 60-70 degrees Fahrenheit.
- Decrease outside noise. Experiment with ear plugs, sleep music, or yoga nidra meditations.
- Decrease the use of electronics, especially in the evening. Blue light affects melatonin release.
- Use blackout curtains or an eye mask; full darkness triggers melatonin.
- Invest in a quality mattress. After all, you spend approximately a third of your life on it!
- Exercise early (this lessens the chance that you won't make excuses throughout the day). Exercise supports sleep.
- Hire a sleep coach—yes, they exist!
- Invest in a heavy or weighted blanket, particularly if you feel anxious.
- Maintain a regular sleep schedule. Routines also aid the sleep cycle.
- Wake up at the same time every day. This creates balanced circadian rhythms.
- Refrain from consuming caffeine in the afternoon. Caffeine is a stimulant.
- Instead, sip hot caffeine-free tea in the afternoon. This creates a calming effect and creates an atmosphere of self-care. Use peppermint tea or its essential oil in water for a pick-me-up!
- Consider taking sleep supplements. Here are some suggestions.
  - Magnesium, which helps regulate the body's stress response system. It fights inflammation, which is the root cause of many diseases. (Additionally, magnesium increases GABA, a neurotransmitter.)
  - GABA encourages relaxation, as well as sleep.
  - 5-HTP (may have side effects).
  - Magnolia Bark.
- Load up on proper amounts of Vitamin D (as D3).

"Sufficient sleep, exercise, healthy food, friendship, and peace of mind are necessities, not luxuries."

– Mark Halperin

VITAMIN D

THE SUNSHINE VITAMIN—VITAMIN D—is so important to our bodies! When properly absorbed, it supports almost all of our body functions and helps to prevent osteoporosis, certain types of cancers, depression, diabetes, and obesity. Vitamin D supports bone health and aids in the absorption of calcium and phosphate from the gastrointestinal tract, as well as cardiovascular and blood sugar balance, musculoskeletal strength, and neurological and immune function.

VITAMIN D IS A CHEERLEADER FOR YOUR BODY!

NOW, SUNLIGHT IS THE OPTIMUM way of getting vitamin D; however, because it is actually difficult to get enough sun exposure and proper absorption, supplementation helps individuals obtain optimal levels.

IN FACT, DEFICIENCY AND INSUFFICIENCY of this nutrient has reached epidemic proportions around the world, leading to more diabetes, multiple sclerosis, rheumatoid arthritis, osteoporosis, breast cancer, prostate cancer, and colon cancer, and other diseases. Depleted levels of vitamin D may interfere with the normal development of teeth and bones, normal cell growth, and contribute to poor regulation of immune and nervous systems.

INDEED, VITAMIN D DEPLETION is problematic, especially in overweight patients with an elevated body mass index—for a poor BMI impairs vitamin D circulation. Absorbing and maintaining vitamin D levels is especially challenging for older patients. Therefore, I recommend D3 for those who have difficulty achieving peak vitamin D levels.

> ***NOTE:** It is important to consult with your physician regarding your current vitamin D levels and whether or not it is necessary to increase or decrease your intake. The normal vitamin D range is between 30-100 ng/ml.*

Vitamin D is also excellent for assisting the digestive system! Let's find out more about digestion. . .

DID YOU KNOW?

It takes about 48 hours for vitamin D to be absorbed from the skin into the body. Washing skin during that time period can interfere with absorption into the blood. Inadequate intake or cholesterol levels can also inhibit the adequate production of the nutrient. Certain medications have been found to contribute to deficiency of vitamin D, including some anti-seizure medications, bile acid sequestrants, oral corticosteroids, and weight loss medications.

DIGESTION DEVELOPMENT

DIGESTION WORKS SO HARD FOR US—let's learn ways to treat it well in return.

HOW THE PROCESS WORKS

THE DIGESTIVE TRACT is a long tube that starts from the mouth and ends in the anus. Once food enters the stomach, it mixes with hydrochloric acid or stomach acids. The stomach also secretes digestive enzymes called pepsin (digests protein) and lipase (digests fat). The stomach turns your food bolus into a liquid called chyme, which passes through the pyloric sphincter to the first part of the small intestine called the duodenum. The gallbladder then releases bile into the duodenum and the pancreas releases certain enzymes to help aid digestion. The small intestine joins with the large intestine, which is where absorption takes place. It is important to note that the small intestine contains finger-like projections on the inside called villi. These create more surface area to help absorb nutrients. Protein and carbohydrates are absorbed directly through the capillary network in our villi and transferred into our bloodstream. These nutrients are then used for growth, energy, and building blocks of our body.

METABOLIC BREAKDOWN OF FOOD

- We consume and digest food. This triggers your metabolism to start working.
- Chyme is the broken-down food that is produced in your stomach.
- Carbohydrates from the food are broken down into simple sugars, also known as glucose.
- Glucose (blood sugar) enters the bloodstream, stimulating insulin production by the pancreas to be transported and distributed throughout the body.
- Insulin, which acts as an usher, opens the door for glucose to enter various cells throughout the body. Some of the glucose is converted into short-term energy for immediate cell usage, while the rest is stored as long-term energy as fat for later use.

> ***NOTE:*** *Digestive enzyme supplementation can be helpful for digestion, as can adding a bitter to your food such as dandelion root.*

ABOUT DIGESTIVE ENZYMES

AS WE AGE, OUR PANCREAS WILL PRODUCE LESS and less digestive enzymes. You will actually find it is harder to digest dinner over breakfast as the pancreas produces less enzymes later in the day.

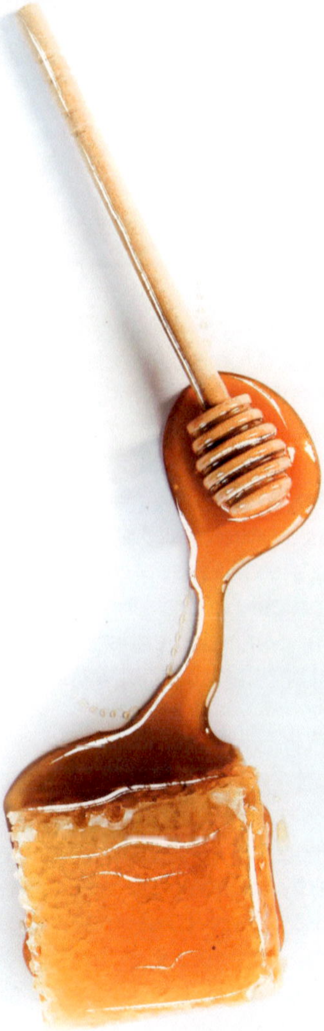

ABOUT PREBIOTICS

PREBIOTICS ARE MOSTLY FIBERS FROM FOOD that stimulate the growth of lactic acid-producing bacteria in the colon. They have been shown to have anti-tumor properties and it will help with the production of vitamin K and B-12 complexes.

PREBIOTICS ALSO STIMULATE the production of probiotics while reducing possible pathogens. They also make the intestinal environment more acidic to enhance mineral absorption.

PLANT FOODS FULL OF PREBIOTICS

- tempeh
- raw pickles
- olives
- green tea
- mushroom
- quinoa
- artichokes
- garlic
- honey
- fruit
- asparagus
- peas
- onions
- legumes
- chicory
- bananas
- burdock root
- chives
- leeks
- kimchi

DID YOU KNOW?

Seventy percent of the immune system is located in your gut and is referred to as gut-associated lymphoid tissue (GALT). It is estimated that the gut contains about 35,000 different strains of bacteria.

PROBIOTICS POWER

CREATE A HEALTHY GUT!

PROBIOTICS ARE LIVE BACTERIA AND YEASTS that are very good for you, especially in terms of keeping the helpful gut bacteria in your digestive system.

The gut is referred to as the place where food is digested, metabolized, and absorbed to be delivered into the cells that provide the body with energy. This process of breaking down food creates bioactive compounds that either help support health or lead to inflammation, which increases the risk of disease.

THE GI TRACT IS A FINELY BALANCED environment where roughly 500 different strains of bacteria compete for space and nutrients. When there is a healthy balance—called eubiosis—few symptoms exist. However, dysbiosis can occur when an overabundance of potentially harmful organisms prevails. The natural microfloral balance can be upset by medications (such as antibiotics or oral contraceptives), excessive alcohol consumption, or poor dietary intake.

PROBIOTICS have been extensively studied and are characterized as having broad GI and immune benefits. The majority are found in the large intestine, particularly the colon, but bacteria can also be found in the esophagus, stomach, and small intestine.

These bacteria serve a variety of functions: hormone rebuilding, promoting healthy metabolism, metabolizing drugs, converting flavonoids to useful forms, and detoxification, which is essential for the removal of waste.

Additionally, they increase the population of healthy bacteria following imbalance of microflora, support healthy bowel function, elevate the production of short-chain fatty acids (providing energy to the cells of the intestinal lining), strengthen the gut-immune barrier by promoting a healthy gut mucosa, and aid in digestion. They even help in breaking down food and difficult-to-breakdown compounds like lactose and casein.

BECAUSE PROBIOTICS ARE LIVE ORGANISMS, there are many challenges associated with manufacturing and distributing probiotic supplements. For a probiotic to be effective, it must be shelf stable through the expiration date and precisely delivered to the intestinal tract, where it can have maximum benefit.

IDEAL ADVICE

TRY 10 OF THE FOLLOWING FOODS FOR AT LEAST ONE WEEK—GET CREATIVE!

Foods That Befriend Digestion:

- avocado
- apple
- blackberries
- bok choy
- broccoli
- brussels sprouts
- cabbage
- cacao
- cantaloupe
- cauliflower
- celery
- chia seeds
- chickpeas
- collard greens
- daikon radishes
- dates
- flax seeds
- ginger
- goji berries
- hemp seeds
- jicama
- peach
- snap peas
- sweet peas
- kale
- mung beans
- nectarine
- raspberries
- pineapple
- sweet potatoes
- okra
- papaya
- sauerkraut
- butternut squash

Foods That Soothe the Stomach:

- ginger
- chamomile
- peppermint
- licorice
- flaxseed
- papaya
- green banana
- pectin (found in apples, citrus, citrus fruits)
- fermented foods
- clear liquids, water

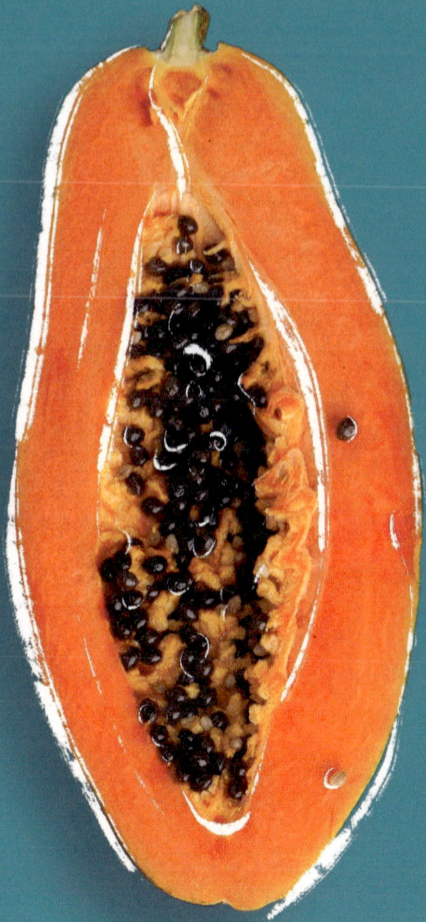

BENEFITS OF PROBIOTICS

- Reduced depression and anxiety.
- Reduced circulating cortisol (called the stress hormone).
- Healthy aging.
- Reduced risk of obesity.
- Increased immune function.
- Stimulated production of short-chain fatty acids, increasing the absorption of calcium, thus reducing oxidative stress.
- Better satiety cues.
- Decreased inflammation.
- Cancer prevention.
- Better detoxification.
- Increased lipid metabolism, decreasing cholesterol.
- Better nutrient utilization.
- More regulated metabolism.
- Reduced recurrent urinary tract infections.
- Manufacturing of B complex and K vitamins.
- Balanced pH levels.
- Lactose and protein digestion.
- Increased absorption of minerals.
- More active peristalsis.
- Regulation of hypertension.

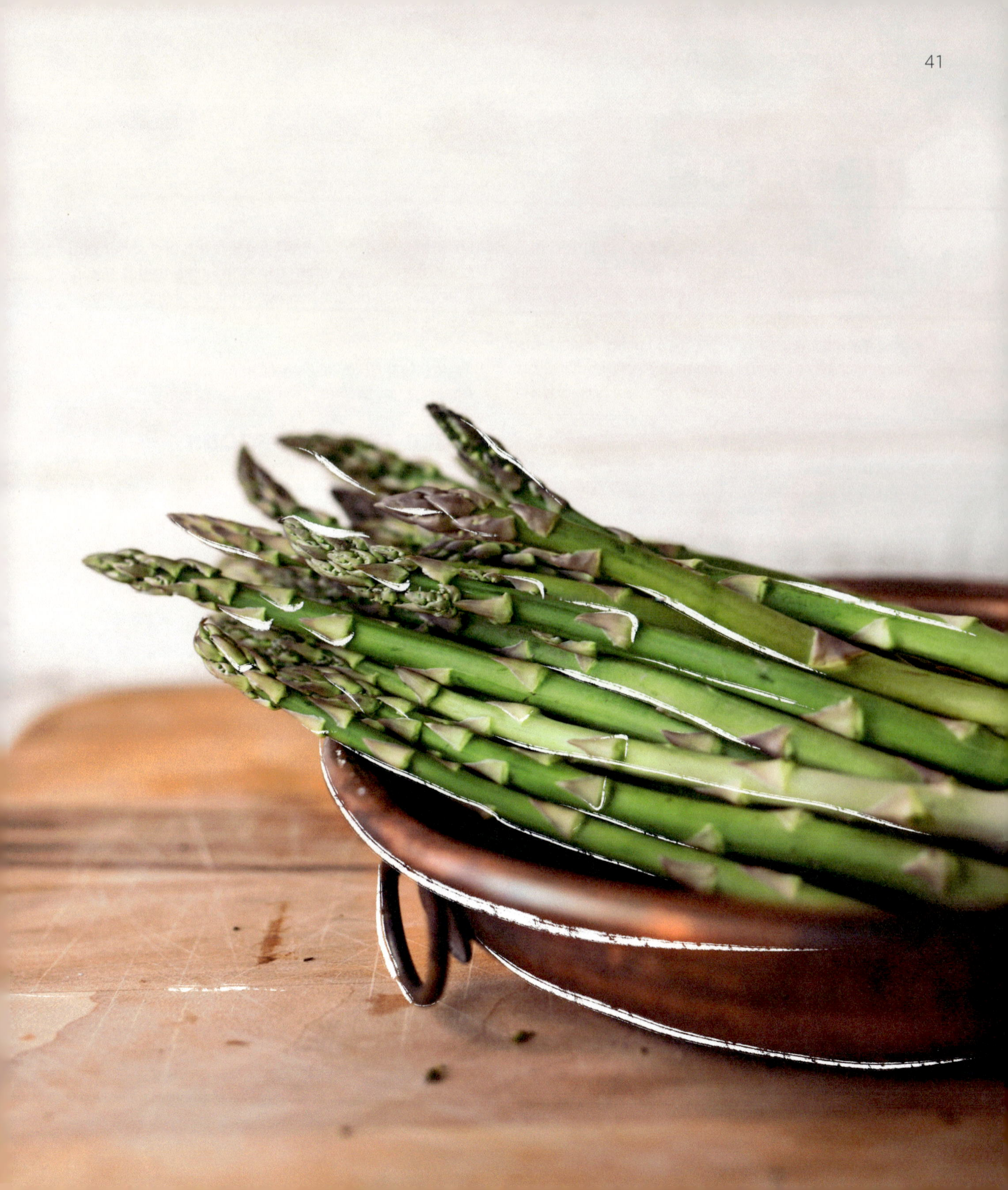

FIBER FUN

FIBER. Not the material that creates your clothes, but the kind that will coat your digestion and clean your colon. When consuming fiber, drink plenty of water, eat fresh fruits and leafy green vegetables, and exercise regularly. Also, avoid using laxatives on a regular basis because they can overstimulate the intestinal muscles and create difficulty with bowel movements.

If you feel gassy or bloated after eating fiber, start with a small amount and increase gradually. A healthy intake of fiber is between 25-45 grams a day, although most Americans do not eat enough fiber. Fiber can improve health in many ways, including promoting intestinal health, decreasing cholesterol, and assisting in weight control.

TYPES OF FIBER

INSOLUBLE FIBERS absorb water to create a soft bulk and helps facilitate the passage of waste products through the intestine at a rapid rate. It can prevent and help treat constipation, diverticulosis, and hemorrhoids. Additionally, it may lower the risk of colon cancer by diluting the effects of harmful substances ingested.

Examples: *rice bran, whole grain, bread, beans, peas, nuts, seeds, and the skins of fruits and vegetables.*

SOLUBLE FIBERS form a gel-like structure that decreases the rate of stomach emptying and absorption of sugars from the intestines. By doing so, it helps control blood sugar levels and lower bad cholesterol. Also, when the stomach empties slowly it helps with weight management by giving you a feeling of fullness.

Examples: *fruits and vegetables, oat bran, barley, beans, peas, prunes, psyllium, flaxseed.*

FIBER-FRIENDLY FOODS

FRUIT AND PORTION:		FIBER IN GRAMS:
• blackberries, 1 cup	=	3.6 g
• bok choy, 1 cup shredded	=	8 g
• brussel sprouts, 1 cup	=	4 g
• chia seeds, 1 oz.	=	10 g
• chickpeas, 1 cup	=	6 g
• almonds, 1 handful	=	4 g
• mung beans, 1 cup	=	8 g
• raspberries, 1 cup	=	8 g
• butternut squash, 1 cup	=	3 g
• sweet peas, 1 cup	=	8 g
• jicama, 1 cup	=	6.5 g
• apple, 1 medium-sized	=	5 g

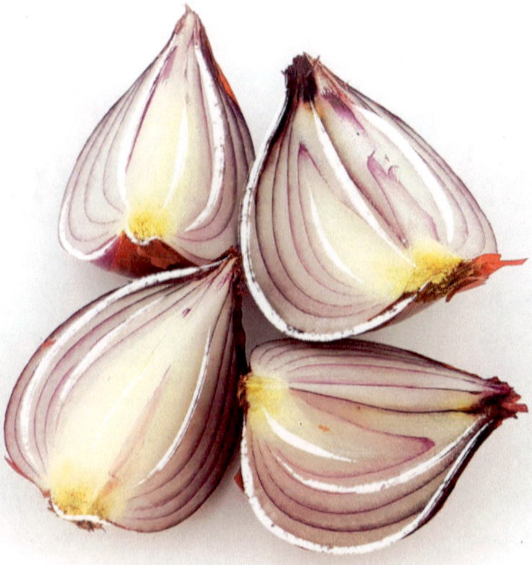

EAT VEGETABLES WITH VIGOR!

WHY ARE VEGETABLES IMPORTANT? Vegetables help to protect your DNA from methylation, an important measurement of cell damage. The more vegetables you consume, the less DNA methylation that occurs, which can help decrease the risk of cancer. Experiment with different ones on different days. Eat them raw, cooked, blended, or juiced on different days—have fun with it!

LOW-CALORIE PLANT FOODS

VEGETABLES (chopped):	CALORIES:	PROTEIN:
red potatoes (1 cup)	108 cal	2.84 g
red onions (1 cup)	67 cal	1.47 g
summer squash (1 cup)	18 cal	1.37 g
mushroom (1 cup)	15 cal	2.16 g
asparagus (1 cup)	27 cal	2.95 g
carrots (1 cup)	52 cal	1.19 g
zucchini (1 cup)	20 cal	1.5 g
brussels sprouts (1 cup)	38 cal	2.97 g
cauliflower (1 cup)	47 cal	2.14 g
butternut squash (1 cup)	63 cal	1.4 g
delicata squash (1 cup)	30 cal	2 g
1 piece of garlic	96 cal	2.25 g
1 sundried tomato	35 cal	1.9 g

IMMUNITY IMPROVEMENTS

WE RELY ON OUR IMMUNE SYSTEM to keep us healthy—we really do. The more "non-ideal" our world becomes, the more we need to boost our immune function!

THINK OF YOUR IMMUNE SYSTEM as an army of cells that defend your body from invaders of any kind, including food, parasites, toxins, bacteria, viruses, and yeast. Your immune system should be able to turn off and on when it is needed and not always operate at the same intensity.

IMMUNITY-BOOSTING FOODS:

- apple cider vinegar
- blueberries
- brazil nuts
- brussels sprouts
- carrots
- cauliflower
- cayenne pepper
- celery
- cilantro
- coconut meat and oil
- daikon radish
- garlic
- ginger
- goji berries
- grapes
- jicama
- scallions
- strawberries
- zucchini

ENJOY THESE OFTEN AND GAIN GREAT ENERGY!

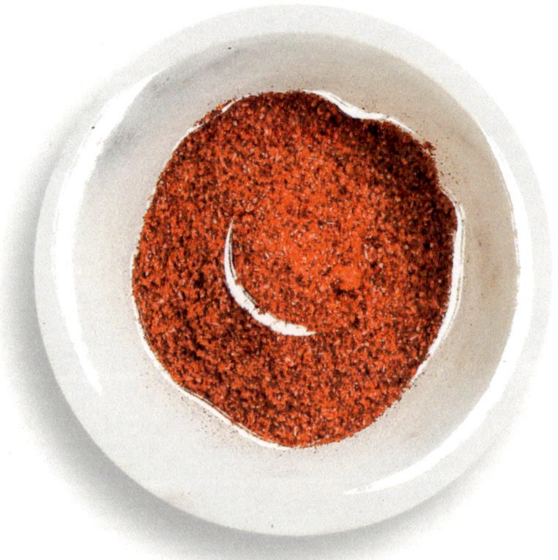

IDEAL ACTION

SUPPORTIVE AFFIRMATIONS

Using the Foods that Boost Immunity list, eat 2-3 of these a day. Work your way down the alphabet!

As you prepare them, say the following affirmations:

I am healthy.

My immune system functions with ease and for my utmost health.

I resist viruses, bacteria, and illness.

My immune system easily wards off dis-ease.

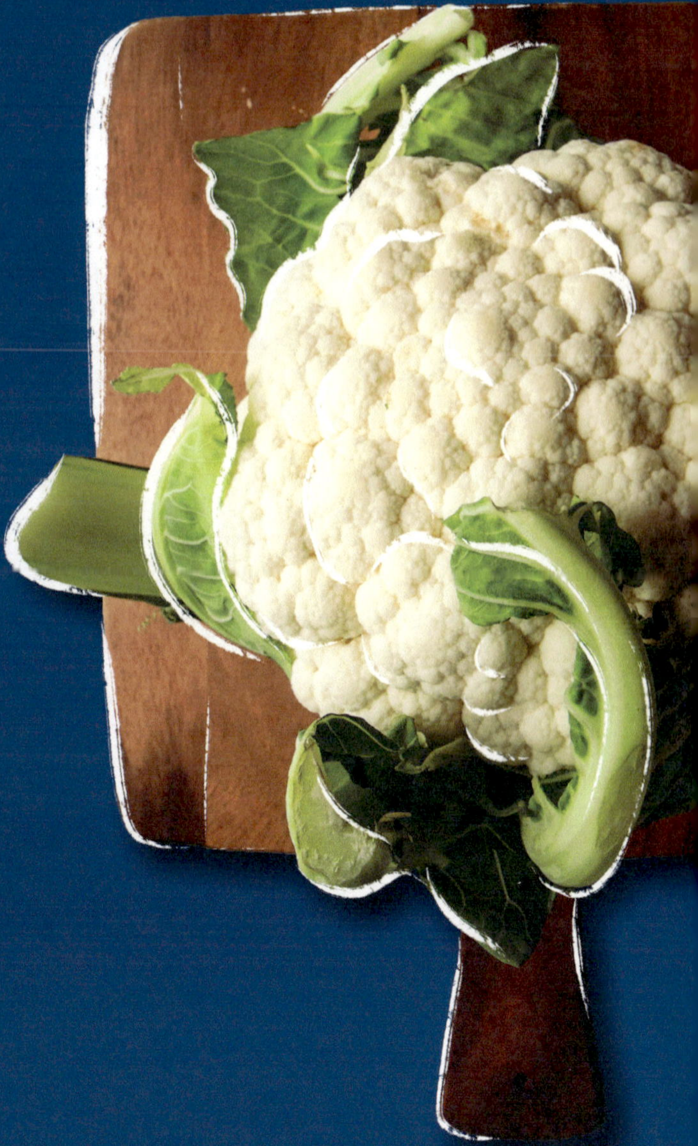

DIALING DETOX

DETOXIFICATION 101

WHY DO DETOX CLEANSING? Well, we live in a toxic world, so periodically we need to clear out and recharge our systems. Here are some reasons.

1. The average woman is exposed to about 126 unique chemical ingredients through using skincare products. Read the label sometime. . . how many of the words sound natural?

2. The average individual is exposed to about 14 pounds of pesticides, herbicides, food additives and preservatives each year.

3. More than 7 million people per year die prematurely from illnesses related to air pollution.

4. It takes approximately 26 seconds for chemicals in typical household products to enter the bloodstream.

5. There are around 80,000 chemicals that have been produced in the world and science is only aware of the effect of 1% - 2% of these! The Environmental Women's Group performed a study on pregnant women and they found over 150 toxins present in the placenta. Just think about what complications these could have on our children.

6. Many foods that we consume can elicit immune reactions that cause weight gain or health issues.

NOW, IN ORDER TO BEGIN YOUR JOURNEY of detoxifying your body, you must also cleanse your mind from toxic thoughts, such as "You are not going to lose weight. No matter what you do, you will just stay like this." One powerful way to counter negativity is to have gratitude in our lives, with thoughts such as, "I am thankful for what I have. I am blessed to have the opportunity to make positive choices, such as going to the grocery store and purchasing ingredients to make a healthy meal to keep my body on the path to wellness."

IDENTIFYING TOXICITY SYMPTOMS

THESE ARE COMMON OUTCOMES OF TOXICITY and signs that you need a detox:

- fatigue
- mental fogginess
- acne
- eczema
- fluctuating levels of energy
- obesity (BMI > 40)
- allergies
- bloating
- heartburn

IDENTIFYING TOXINS

ENVIRONMENTAL TOXINS:

- pollution (air, water, ground)
- auto exhaust

- solvents
- occupational hazards
- heavy metals, mercury fillings
- pesticides, herbicides, insecticides
- radiation, UV light

"LIFESTYLE" TOXINS:

- fast and fried foods
- processed food and preservatives
- cosmetics
- nicotine
- prescription drugs
- meats containing hormones and antibiotics
- refined sugars

FOOD TOXINS AKA TOP ALLERGENS:

- eggs
- milk
- fish
- peanuts
- pork
- gluten
- shellfish
- soy
- tree nuts
- wheat
- corn

THE DETOX PROCESS

DETOXIFYING ORGANS

1. Liver: Elimination. As the liver has perhaps the most complex detoxification process, there are some theories on the best method to enhance this pathway. Studies show that it causes the release of fat-soluble toxins into the colon for elimination and allows the liver to create more glutathione.

2. Kidneys: Excretion. The kidneys are the pathway for eliminating water-soluble toxins that have passed through the liver.

3. Intestines: Excretion. Also, fat tissue around the stomach causes secretion of interleukins from white blood cells, which can cause disease due to inflammation. This is another reason why weight loss is important. Although there is some controversy surrounding colon hydrotherapy (colonics), it is suggested that it helps with body detoxification.

4. Skin: Sweating. Through the skin—our largest organ—is how we sweat out toxins in our bodies. This can be done through exercising or using various types of saunas or steam rooms at levels that you are able to tolerate.

DID YOU KNOW?

Though rich in important amino acids, whey protein is derived from milk and can cause inflammation. There are other more organic forms of whey (i.e. fortified isolate and hydrolyzed whey), however, I recommend refraining from any form of whey during the detox period.

NATURAL DETOX FOODS & HERBS

THERE ARE CERTAIN FOODS, HERBS, AND DRINKS that aid in the process of liver detoxification. Here is a list below:

- turmeric
- broccoli
- green tea
- spinach
- kale
- chlorella
- rice bran
- fiber

AFTER DETOX, YOUR PALATE SENSITIVITY will change. As a result, your lifestyle will change; you will be led to behavioral changes that you will enjoy for the long term and not cause feelings of being deprived. Toxins cause many diseases and health issues, such as obesity.

Now, I did my detox using a powder that has brown rice protein, gentle fiber, and a unique blend of nutrients and vegetables that protect against cell damage and induce the expression of glutathione. I must admit that I felt tired during the first day, but on day two, I began to feel more energetic and noticed that my cravings were decreasing.

During a cleanse, symptoms vary with different individuals, as some may experience a mild headache and/or nausea during the first couple of days (due to their past unhealthy diet and sugar withdrawal). Others may not experience any of these symptoms at all.

ALSO, ALKALINE FOODS ARE IMPORTANT. If you do not consume enough alkaline foods, your body draws it from weaker bones. Acid- forming foods take calcium from the bones and becomes the main reason for osteoporosis. Synthetic drugs, meat, dairy, and white flour contribute to calcium deficiency, whereas dark greens like kale are examples of foods containing alkaline.

DID YOU KNOW?

Small amounts of cyanide are found in nature and in some foods we eat. Spinach has trace amounts, so it's best to bring the water to boil, throw the spinach in and let it steam for one minute. Remove the water, use what you need, and freeze the rest in small containers for later use. Unfreeze a day in advance. This process should remove the toxins.

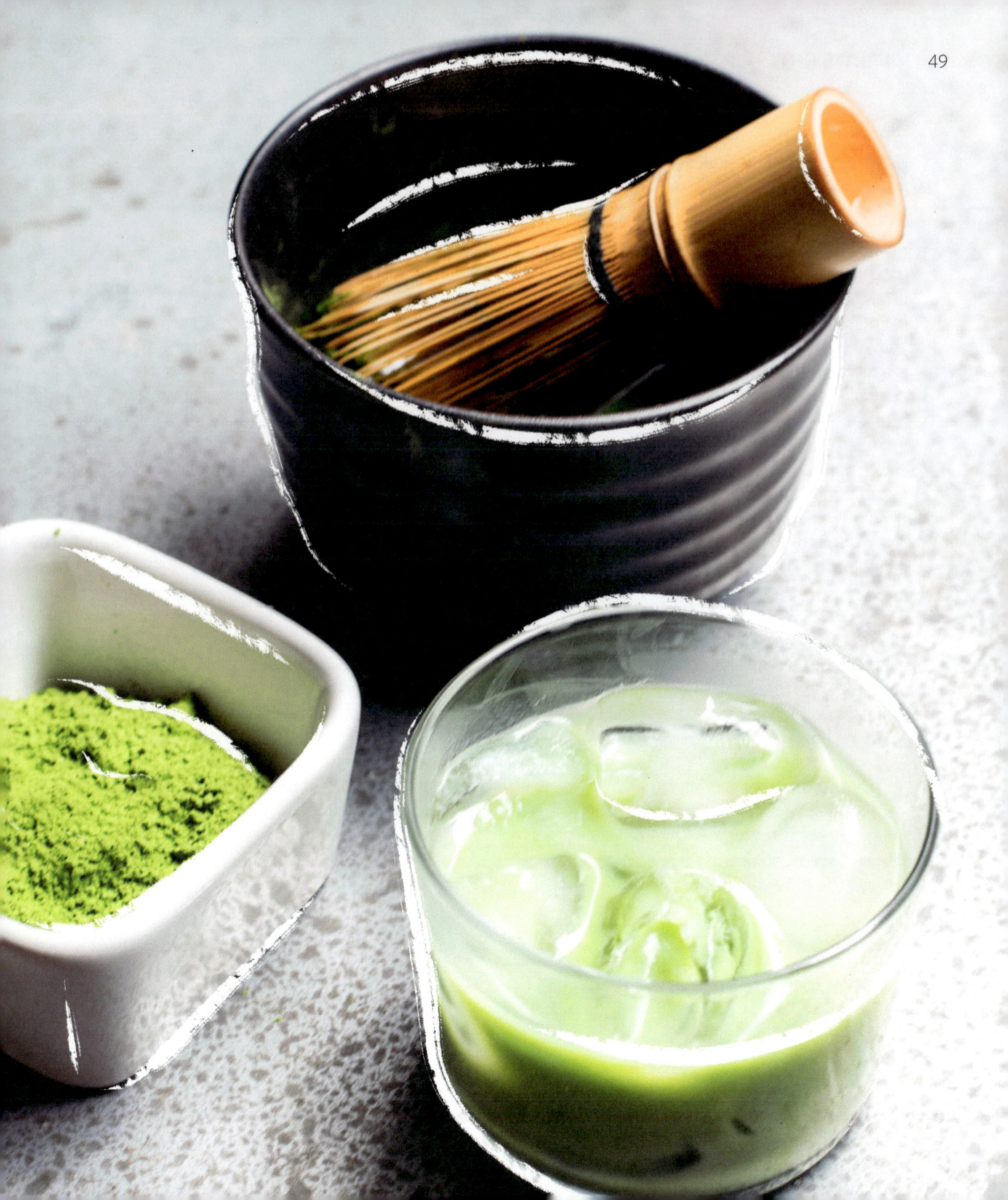

ELIMINATION DIET

AN ELIMINATION DIET IS WHEN YOU TAKE AWAY foods that you may be allergic to. Eliminating toxic foods slowly from your diet can be done anywhere from 3 weeks to 3 months. Simply remove it from your cooking routine and know that usually there is a healthy replacement. Notice if you feel less bloated, less gas, better bowel movements, or have more energy.

Upon completing your elimination diet, you can add one food item at a time back into your diet to observe whether or not your old toxicity symptoms return. Watch for rashes, stomach pain, fatigue, painful joints, bloating, or a change in bowel habits.

THEN, DO A 3-4 DAY ROTATIONAL DIET, where you do not consume the same foods everyday, as this can allow you to assess what foods your body can tolerate. For example, you may have potatoes on Monday, but not again until Friday. Then see how you feel.

You must change some of harmful things in your life that were comfortable in order to take important steps toward healthy lifestyle changes! Remember that sometimes the food you crave is actually the food you are allergic to.

FOODS TO ELIMINATE

- Gluten, dairy, soy.
- Strawberries. Hard to believe it can be harmful, but depends on your constitution.
- Eggs. Eliminate for the first 2 weeks, then reintroduce; wait 72 hours to record how you feel.
- Yeast. It is often bothersome.
- Corn. It is a very common irritant.
- Nightshade vegetables. Remove eggplant, peppers, potatoes, and tomatoes.
- Sesame seeds. Even these can be troublesome!

REPLACEMENT SUGGESTIONS

- Try plant-based protein smoothies instead of yogurt-based ones.
- Make steamed vegetables, kale, spinach, and collard greens instead of nightshades.
- Use sweet potatoes instead of potatoes.
- Have slow cooked brown rice (gluten-free) instead of bread.
- Enjoy adzuki and mung beans instead of soy.

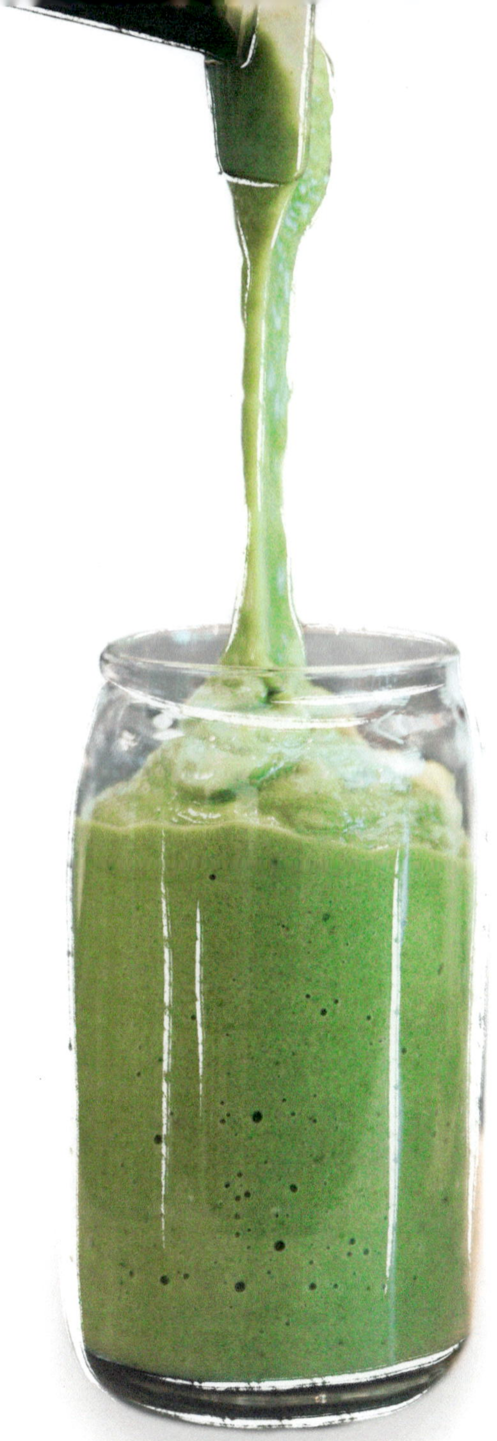

IDEAL ACTION

Take your food journal and turn it in a "symptom diary" for additional support. Write down how you are feeling after eating certain foods. You will become aware of what foods affect you.

DECELERATE DIABETES

DIABETES: *THE MOTHER OF DISEASES.* Why risk one day being diagnosed with diabetes when you could simply change your lifestyle?

WHAT IS YOUR RISK?

IF YOU HAVE ANY OF THESE INDICATORS listed below, finding and maintaining your ideal weight is even more important. At least two of these factors increase the risk of developing type 2 diabetes.

- A history of prediabetes.
- A family history of diabetes.
- Being of African American, Latino American, Asian American, Native American, or Pacific Islander descent.
- Having had gestational diabetes (diabetes during pregnancy).
- Being over the age of 45.
- Obesity and a large waist size (35 inches for women and 40 inches for men).
- Doing little or no physical activity.
- Having hypertension.
- Having low levels of good cholesterol (HDL).
- Having elevated triglycerides (fat in the blood).

SYMPTOMS OF DIABETES

Some people might have diabetes without exhibiting any symptoms.

By living an Ideal Weights lifestyle, you can do your best to avoid a lifetime of managing these debilitating symptoms.

- Frequent urination.
- Extreme thirst.
- Unusual hunger.
- Extreme fatigue.
- Blurred vision.
- Skin infections that are slow to heal.
- Tingling or numbness in the feet.

COMPLICATIONS *IDENTIFIED BY THE CENTER FOR DISEASE CONTROL*

HEALTH RISKS OF HAVING DIABETES

- 2-3 times the rate of death from heart disease.
- 2-4 times higher risk of stroke.

DID YOU KNOW?

THESE ARE LOW-GLYCEMIC FRUITS:

- apple
- blackberries
- blueberries
- cherries
- nectarine
- pear
- peaches
- pink grapefruit
- plums
- pomegranate
- raspberries
- strawberries
- red grapes

- Having high blood pressure. Over 70% of people with diabetes have high BP.
- Becoming blind.
- Suffering from neuropathy. Between 60-70 % of diabetics suffer from mild to severe nervous system damage.
- Possible amputation. Over 60% of all lower limb amputations occur with diabetes.
- Increased chance of end-stage kidney disease.
- Increased frequency and severity of gum disease and dental health issues that can lead to eventual tooth loss.
- Pregnancy complications.
- Increased susceptibility to other illnesses and death.

PREDIABETES FAST FACTS *FROM THE CENTER FOR DISEASE CONTROL*

A total of 84.1 million adults, 18 years or older, are prediabetic (33.9% of the adult population) and approximately 23.1 million adults aged 65 years or older have prediabetes. An estimated 30.3 million people have diabetes (9.4% of the US population), while there are about 7.2 million individuals who have undiagnosed diabetes.

IDEAL ADVICE

DIABETIC EATING TIPS

- Maintain a healthy weight.
- Consume foods high in fiber. They are satiating as well.
- Enjoy low-glycemic foods. These are slower acting carbohydrates and more satiating.
- Eat more foods with unsaturated fats. Examples include avocado and avocado oil, olives and olive oil, almond butter, nuts and seeds (like almonds and sesame).
- Eat whole grains in small portions.
- Fill ½ of your plate with vegetables, such as broccoli, green beans, and collard greens.
- Fill ¼ of your plate with plant-based protein. Examples include chickpeas, red lentils, a variety of beans, lentils, spirulina, quinoa, green peas, and edamame.
- Use hemp seeds and spirulina on your plate.
- Fill the last ¼ of your plate with whole grains (quinoa, wild rice, oats, bulgar).
- Drink water ½ an hour before or 45 minutes after a meal. Avoid drinking any liquids with your meal.

HONING HYPERTENSION

LET'S BEAT HYPERTENSION! Also known as high blood pressure (BP), it can lead to many complications including those associated with diabetes, such as diabetic eye disease and kidney disease. Most people with diabetes will eventually develop high blood pressure, along with other heart and circulation problems.

GUIDELINES *established by the American Heart Association (for adults ages 18 and older).*

SYSTOLIC BP

Normal: below 120
Prehypertension: 120-129
Hypertension stage 1:130-139
Hypertension stage 2: 140 or higher

DIASTOLIC BP

Normal: below 80
Prehypertension: below 80
Hypertension stage 1: 80-89
Hypertension stage 2: 90 or higher

Stage 1 hypertension can be treated with lifestyle changes, however, stage 2 hypertension typically requires drug intervention in conjunction with lifestyle changes. Chronic hypertension increases the workload of the heart, causing damage to arteries. This damage, in turn, creates arteriosclerosis, thus increasing the risk of heart disease. Treating hypertension early can decrease the risk of acquiring certain heart diseases later on.

TREATING BP WITHOUT MEDICATION

- Monitor salt intake, as salt increases blood pressure. If using salt, choose pink Himalayan salt. Himalayan salt contains 84 minerals and trace minerals, such as calcium, copper, iron, magnesium, and potassium, giving the salt its slight pink tint. Still, be sure to monitor any amount or type you consume.

- Eat adequate amount of fruits and green leafy vegetables.

- Lose weight if overweight.

- Limit or avoid alcohol.

- Avoid smoking.

- Exercise regularly.

"IT IS HEALTH THAT IS REAL WEALTH AND NOT PIECES OF GOLD AND SILVER." -MAHATMA GANDHI

KNOW YOUR ABC'S

High blood pressure and high cholesterol are risk factors of diabetes and can lead to other chronic health problems.

A=HEMOGLOBIN. A1c reflects your average blood glucose over a 3-month period. Suggested target = below 6.

B=BLOOD PRESSURE. When it is too high, it causes your heart to pump harder in order to perfuse all organs in the body. Suggested target = below 130/80.

C=CHOLESTEROL. Bad cholesterol (called LDL) can build up and clog your arteries. Suggested target = below 100.

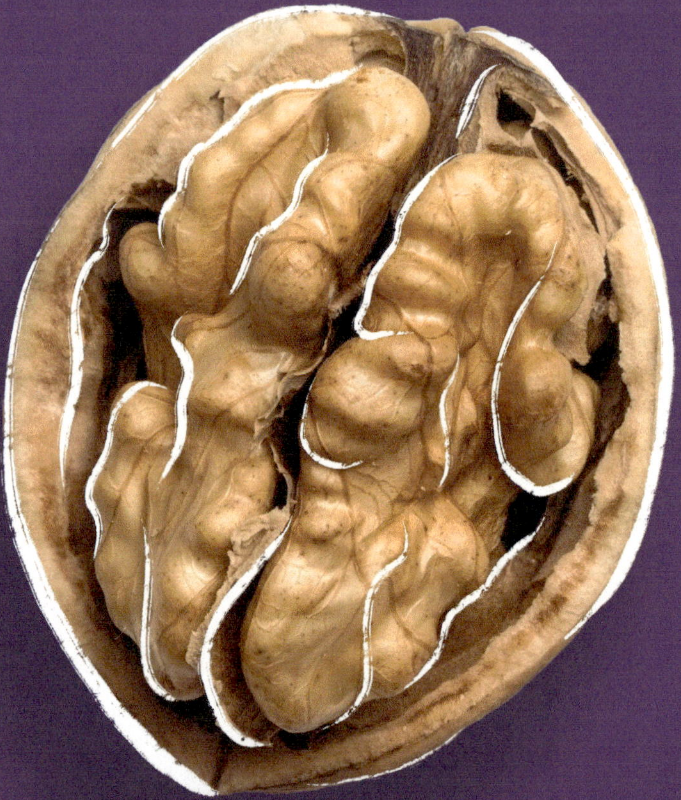

“KNOWLEDGE IS THE FOOD OF THE SOUL.”

-PLATO

STAY IN THE KNOW

AN IMPORTANT ASPECT OF MAINTAINING GOOD health pertains to making informed decisions regarding nutrition. When eating clean, you're much more likely to keep your caloric intake at an appropriate level for your body and maintain a healthy weight as a result.

WHOLE FOODS WILL SATISFY and keep you full, whereas empty calories (like those found in candy and chips) offer a quick boost of energy, but often lead to a crash and a return of hunger shortly after.

HERE ARE TIPS AND "TRANSLATIONS" for *really* reading food labels, as well as understanding more about foods and sources that are "not so clean."

FOOD LABEL INTERPRETATION

AS DEFINED BY THE FOOD AND DRUG ADMINISTRATION. Learn how to read labels to stay properly informed.

"Low" calories = 40 calories or less.

"Light" = fewer calories or 50% or less fat than the regular product.

"Fat-free" = less than ½ a gram of fat.

"Low" fat = 3 grams or less of fat.

"Reduced" fat = 25% less than the regular product.

"Fewer or fewer calories" = at least 25% fewer calories than the regular product.

"INDULGE" FOOD INFORMATION

FOOD:	FAT:	CALORIES:
small cut fries (2 oz.)	15 g	265
1 large french fry	25 g	500
potato chips (3 oz.)	30 g	450
cola (8 fl oz.)		100
(12 fl oz.)		150
(1 L)		400
(2 L)		800

NOTE: *Products labeled as having "zero grams of trans fat" are still high in fat and calories! For instance, take the example of Lay's barbecue chips: one, 7-ounce bag contains 972 calories. It also contains 64.15 grams of fat. Despite this, the bag is labeled as having zero grams of trans fat.*

Make sure to read all labels carefully.

FOODS TO KNOW MORE ABOUT

FOODS THAT LOWER LDL (BAD CHOLESTEROL):

- almonds
- apple
- avocado
- cabbage
- chickpeas
- grapefruit
- hemp seeds
- kale
- olive oil
- pine nuts
- pistachios
- sunflower seeds
- turmeric

FAT

FATS ARE USED AS RESERVED FUEL. High blood glucose (sugars) elicits the release of insulin, causing cell tissues to uptake glucose and favor the storage of fuels as glycogen and triglycerides, while also aiding in the immobilization of fatty acids in adipose tissue.

TWO TYPES OF FATS

Healthy fats: avocados, seeds, nuts, olive oil.

Unhealthy fats: animal fats, chips, fried foods.

All fats that you consume will eventually build up into the cell membrane. For a moment, imagine these cell membranes being composed of potato chips and bacon. Unhealthy fats actually change the structure of our cell membrane, making them stiff and rigid. This change in their composition causes them to damage the body, including plaque formation in the arteries. Ideally, we want healthy fats to help our cells move more fluidly through the bloodstream and allowing transport of nutrients across the cell membrane with ease.

GLUTEN

INDEED, GLUTEN IS RESPONSIBLE for the elastic texture of dough. It has a protein called glutamorphine that are morphine-like peptides, which cause addiction. Gluten is in cereal grains, wheat flour, and dough.

Gluten triggers an autoimmune response that attacks the lining of the small intestine in people who are intolerant, such as those with Celiac disease. This disrupts the body's ability to absorb nutrients into the bloodstream properly, leading to anemia, delayed growth, and unwanted weight loss. Approximately 1 in 33 people in the United States have Celiac disease. Gluten is also known to cause other illnesses besides Celiac disease.

GLUTEN-FREE FOODS:

- potatoes
- buckwheat
- oats (must be labeled GF)
- corn
- rice
- quinoa
- amaranth
- teff
- millet
- beans
- nuts and nut butters
- eggs
- fresh fruits
- fresh vegetables
- herbs and spices
- meat and fish
- juice (100% natural)
- homemade soups (no bouillon cubes due to malt)

DAIRY

HUMANS ARE THE ONLY SPECIES that consume milk in adulthood. In fact, about 75% of the world's population is unable to break down lactose. The main carbohydrate in milk is lactose and it is composed of two simple sugars: glucose and galactose. As an infant, your body produces a digestive enzyme called lactase, which breaks down lactose from your mother's milk. Many people lose their ability to break down lactose in adulthood.

It can take 10 days to 3 weeks to eliminate cow's milk protein from your system, so you need at least 3 weeks of elimination before evaluating the results.

Dairy contains large amounts of saturated fat, which is linked to heart disease and can cause digestive issues and excess mucus. Conjugated linoleic acid and fatty chain amino acids found in dairy may contribute to slowing the breakdown of fat. Fermented or pasteurized dairy products are less damaging. Try hemp, almond, or rice milks, and cashew cheeses instead

I avoid dairy because it is often full of hormones meant for animals—and fats like dairy create more hunger cues. Fatty foods like cheese keep your hunger center open.

DAIRY DRAWBACKS

- **SKIN SENSITIVITY.** A high consumption of full-fat dairy may increase the risk of developing moderate to severe acne—particularly among teens.
- **DIGESTIVE DISTRESS.** Many who consume milk are unaware that this habit may be causing digestive issues. A large percentage of Asian Americans, Native Americans, and African Americans encounter gastrointestinal cramping, flatulence, and diarrhea. Some may also find that they have a harder time tolerating dairy as they age.
- **CANCER CONCERNS.** The Physician Health Study—one of the largest running studies on men's health—concluded that men who consumed high levels of dairy had a significant risk for developing prostate cancer.
- **CONTAMINANTS CHALLENGE.** Synthetic hormones like recombinant bovine growth hormone (rBGH) are often given to cows to increase dairy production. As a result, these hormones make their way into our milk supply. The same goes for antibiotics administered to animals that develop infections due to milk production manipulation. Please limit your intake of diary whenever possible!

DID YOU KNOW?

Dairy was not consumed by humans until after the agricultural revolution.

NOTE: *Farm-raised animals often suffer in terrible conditions and are abused. They are in tightly cramped quarters and are barely able to move. Animal products are high in omega-6 that they get from being fed grains. Too much omega-6 raises your blood pressure and can lead to blood clots, heart attacks, strokes, and water retention.*

SUPPLEMENT SUPPORT

EVERYTHING, INCLUDING THE FOOD WE EAT, is a supplement. Because supplements are not regulated by the Food and Drug Administration, there are concerns about mislabeling, compromised quality, and the potential for adverse side effects.

There are many aspects to consider regarding supplements; since daily nutritional intake has a significant impact, it is ideal to first practice understanding how to eat well and then consider adding supplements.

WHILE MULTIPLE STUDIES VALIDATE that supplements aid in nutrient absorption for the prevention of chronic diseases—thus increasing lifespan—other studies negate these findings.

Generally, supplements are often useful for people who are unable to obtain adequate nutrition from their diet alone. For example, vegans are recommended to take vitamin B-12 supplements, as B-12 comes from red meat.

NOTE: *I recommend rotating supplements and taking them on different days. Observe how you feel without taking them and then scale back to the basics. Too much supplementation can be like taking unnecessary medications.*

However, since we live in a toxic and polluted world, we need the support of supplements!

SIGNS OF A DEFICIT:

- chronic fatigue
- digestive issues
- lowered immunity
- hair loss
- clouded consciousness
- long term veganism
- fallout from a high-stress lifestyle

If you have any of the above, work with your physician to see if a supplement regimen can help alleviate your symptoms. Make sure you purchase high-quality vitamins. Once you create this habit, you will be grateful for the changes that occur!

Keep in mind, just because a supplement has made it to the store shelves and is being sold does *not* make it a quality product.

RECOMMENDED FOR DAILY USE:

- multi-vitamins
- vitamin D3
- natural fish oils
- co-enzyme Q10
- probiotics
- B-12
- calcium

These are crucial to the body systems, create basic health, and can be taken regularly. However, while supplements are meant to help "encourage" a healthy diet and should always be taken under a physician's supervision, some may cause adverse reactions.

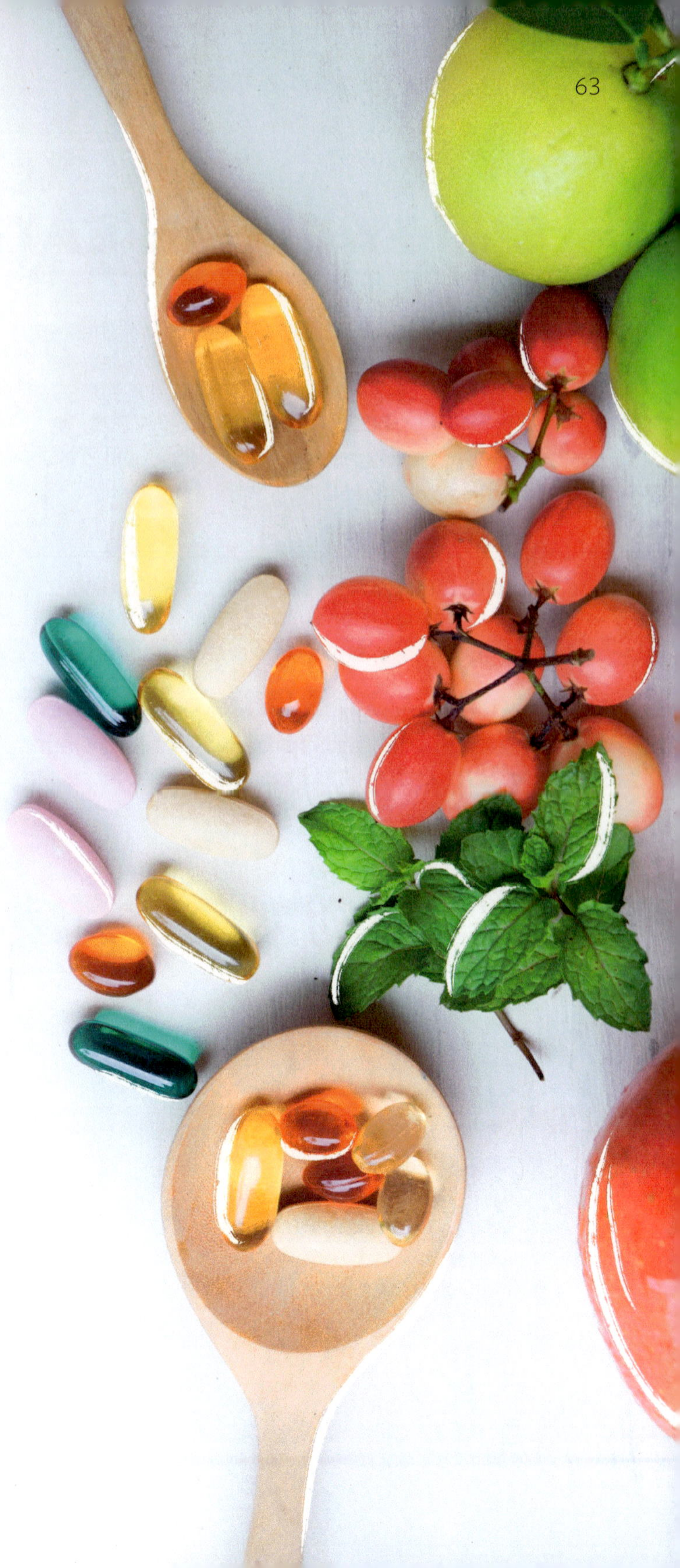

ENJOY CLEAN EATING

YOU MAY FIND THROUGH CLEAN EATING that you begin to engage in other healthy lifestyle changes. If you practice Clean Eating, you may find it easier to also engage in self-care practices such as exercise, meditation, massages, and other techniques that help make your life rich and vibrant.

WHEN YOU FEEL GREAT, YOU ARE ABLE to move throughout the day with more joy and ease, as well as create supportive and nurturing relationships in your career and with your family.

Ever since I made the choice to eat clean, my outlook on life has changed noticeably. I have more energy to do the things I like to do; I read more and am more focused. This book is another positive outcome of my journey!

EMPOWER YOURSELF WITH KNOWLEDGE and make the best choices for heath—and for yourself.

BENEFITS OF CLEAN EATING

- Clear skin.
- Weight loss.
- Increased energy.
- Stronger hair and nails.
- Improved sleep.
- Less exposure to chemicals.
- Less exposure to hormones.
- Regulation of cholesterol.
- Cancer prevention.
- Decreased risk of dementia.
- Improved overall digestive system.
- Natural intake of vitamins and minerals.

IMPLEMENTING CLEAN EATING

1. Consume whole foods that are minimally processed. Avoid unrecognized, chemical ingredients and packaged foods. If you are not vegetarian or vegan, eat pasture-raised, grass-fed and free-range meats and eggs. Nuts and seeds should be used in small quantities.

2. Experiment with home cooking. Restaurant grade food is typically not the best quality and has a variety of preservatives and unhealthy additives. Keep it simple until you acquire more knowledge about other recipes.

3. Never cook with extra virgin olive oil. It has a very low melting point, meaning it will burn fast at 200-250 degrees Farenheit. Avocado oil is a better option. Do not cook your food for too long, as studies suggest that 50-80% of nutrients are lost by doing so. Decrease cooking time to preserve the nutrients.

4. Limit refined carbohydrates, including white sugar, white flour, white rice, pasta, pastries, and bread.

5. Maintain consistent eating times.

6. Balance your plate. Aim to consume protein, a small number of carbohydrates and healthy fats at every meal. This will create optimal blood sugar levels and will assist with satiation to reduce cravings.

7. Enjoy non-starchy vegetables, particularly ones grown above the ground: leafy greens, cabbage, broccoli, and cauliflower.

8. Have low-sugar fruits like avocado, cucumber, olives, and berries.

9. Integrate eating fermented foods: sauerkraut, kimchi, pickles, kefir (with a coconut-based milk), and small amounts of high-quality kombucha.

IDEAL ACTION

As a start to eating clean and healthy, begin by adding one unprocessed food item to your diet twice a month, preferably an item of food that you have never purchased before. By the end of the year, you will have added multiple unprocessed foods to your diet, thus creating sustainable lifestyle changes. Here are some examples of foods to incorporate.

Plant-based protein sources: legumes, tempeh, beans.

Healthy fat options: avocado, olive oil, nuts, seeds.

Complex carbohydrates: whole grains, brown rice, buckwheat.

Vegetables: sweet potato, brussels sprouts, artichokes.

"TO EAT IS A NECESSITY, BUT TO EAT INTELLIGENTLY IS AN ART."

– FRANCOIS DE LA ROCHEFEOUCAULD

FOOD COMBINING

PROPER FOOD COMBINING IS A WELL-TESTED way to understand optimum eating and efficient digesting.

WHEN YOU COMBINE FOODS with varying cooking times (like raw fruit with meats), digestive problems may ensue. For example, if you had a meal that included pineapple and shrimp, the fruit sits in the stomach much longer than it would if it was being eaten alone. As a result, the sugars in the fruit ferment, which leads to bloating and gas. This problem will multiply from there and cause malabsorption of all of its nutrients.

Anytime there is fermentation from poor food combining, it can create gas that is toxic and even carcinogenic. As a result, you may feel fatigued, experience inflammation, constipation, arthritis, colitis, high blood pressure, and other unpleasant issues.

Also, any liquid taken with your food in your stomach dilutes the enzymes your body needs to digest protein, carbs, and fats. Water goes through your stomach in about 10 minutes, while juices take about 15-30 minutes. However, taken 45 minutes post any meal, water rinses and hydrates the tract, fiber sweeps and cleanses, and enzymes activate the chemical process of digestion.

PROPER FOOD COMBINING truly makes a difference. Pay attention to this information and give these instructions a shot. You will be amazed at the results.

WHAT TO EAT WHEN

1. Listen to your body. Your first meal of the day is very important.

2. Eat only when you are hungry and chew slowly. When you are full, stop eating.

3. Refrain from eating dairy, gluten, and sugar.

4. Eat fruit 30-60 minutes before your meals, it will prepare the digestive tract with enzyme stimulation. On average, fruits take 30-60 minutes to digest.

5. After a meal, wait at least 3 hours before eating fruits.

8. Vegetables, grains, and beans take 1-2 hours to digest.

9. Cooked meat and fish take at least 3-4 hours to digest.

10. Shellfish takes 4-8 hours to digest.

11. Consuming more fiber in your diet can help you to feel full, thus reducing the onset of cravings.

12. Eat plant-based protein. If you do eat animal protein, have no more than 3-4 ounces a day of organic or grass-fed.

IDEAL ADVICE

FOOD SHOPPING & PREPARATION TIPS

- Do not shop hungry!
- Plan your menu ahead of time in order to build a shopping list and then refrain from going to the store without it.
- Spend money on quality ingredients. Buy organic, local, and in-season as much as possible.
- Buy in bulk, either directly from the farmer or at discount stores. Eating foods that are not packaged are less processed.
- Stay away from whey protein, dairy, and gluten. See replacement suggestions and enjoy new things!
- Shop from the perimeter of the grocery store, as these areas have fresh fruits and vegetables. The center aisles typically contain more processed foods.
- Read the labels carefully. The first four ingredients are the most important part of the products. RULE: If you cannot pronounce it, stay away from it.
- Experiment with growing your own vegetables, fruits, and herbs.
- Keep a well-stocked kitchen. This limits poor decisions like eating comfort food or spontaneous eating out.
- Take a few hours out of your day off and prepare your food for the week. Being organized will help you stick to your healthy eating plan.
- Make meal planning and preparation a "family affair." Make it fun! Plan theme nights (i.e. Meatless Monday, Lentil Wednesday, Salad Saturday).

IDEAL ACTION

MAKE MEAL PLANS FOR A MONTH

Use these recommended ingredients to plan your meals for a month. Remember, home cooking is cheaper, more nutritious and fresh, and offers minimally-processed foods, fewer additives, and less packaging waste. But, do not cook your food for too long. Scientific studies show that you lose 50-80% of the nutrients. So, cook al denté to preserve most of the nutrients. Here are ingredient ideas for proper planning.

- Week 1 Antioxidant foods:
  - beans, berries, broccoli, cantaloupe, cauliflower, garlic, ginger, nuts, papaya, spinach, snow peas, sweet potatoes, turnip greens
- Week 2 Immune-enhancing foods:
  - apples, asparagus, broccoli, cayenne pepper, cherries, cilantro, ginger, goji berries, green tea, red and yellow onions, turmeric
- Week 3 Anti-inflammatory foods:
  - arugula, bell peppers, blackberries, blueberries, cabbage, cacao, cantaloupe, cauliflower, cilantro, radishes
- Week 4 Anti-aging foods:
  - avocado, blueberries, broccoli, dark chocolate, edamame, green leafy vegetables, green tea, nuts, pomegranates, sweet potatoes, watermelon

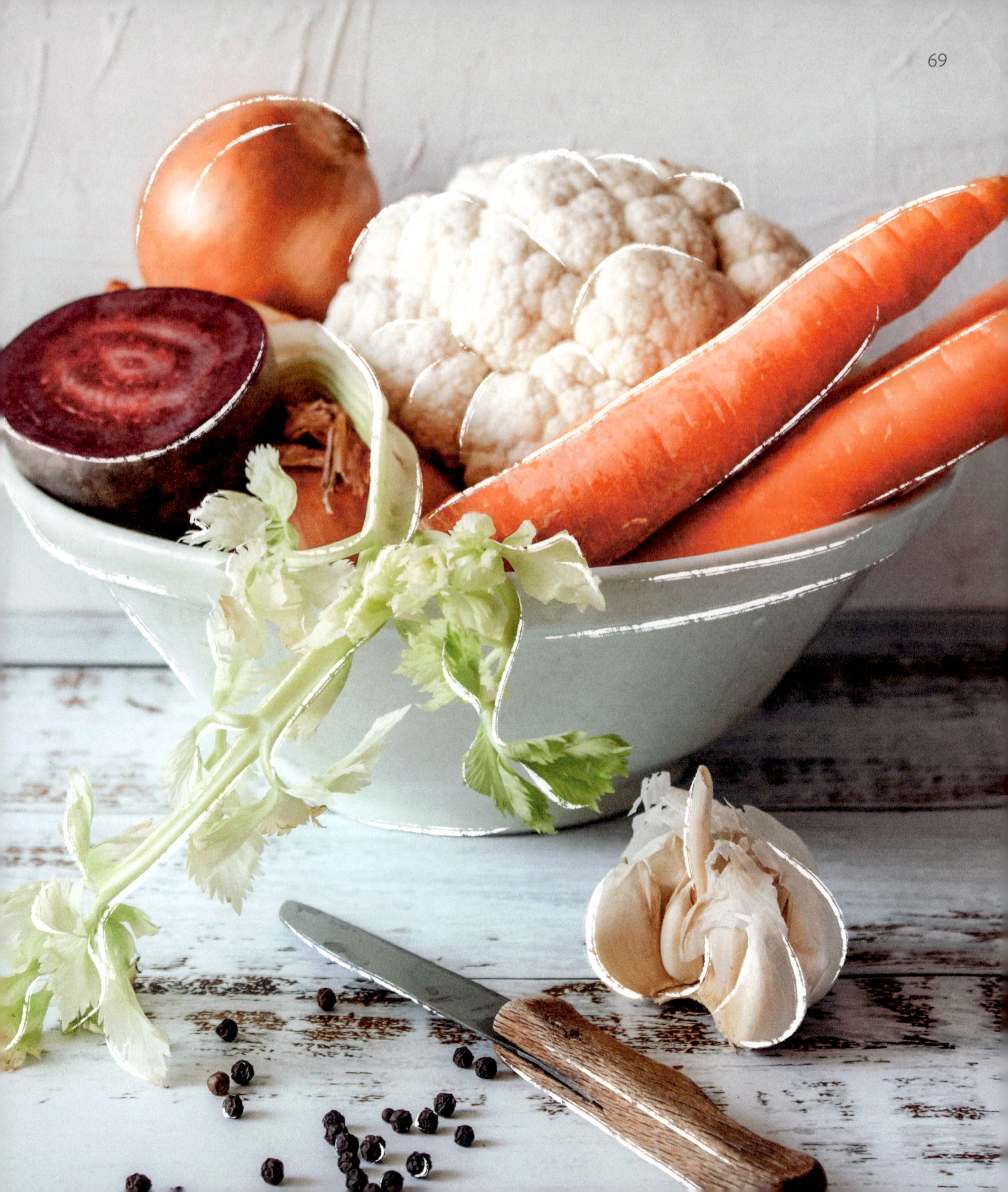

“FIND A PLACE
THERE IS JOY,
WILL BURN OUT
-JOSEPH

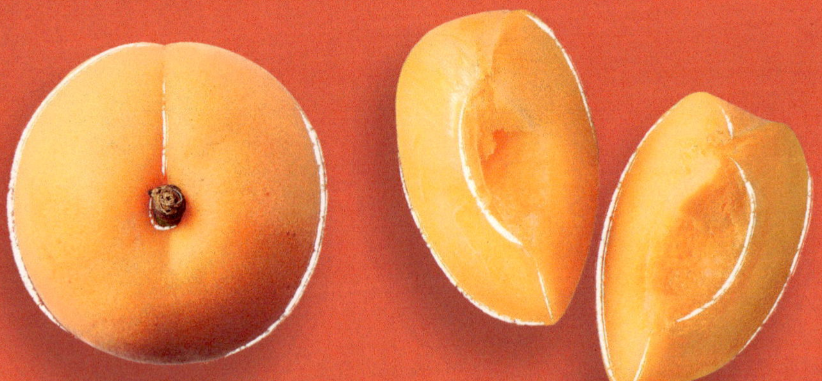

INSIDE WHERE

AND THE JOY

THE PAIN."

CAMPBELL

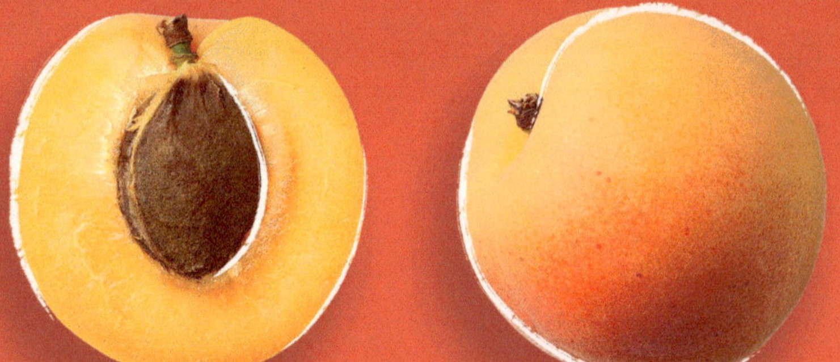

KNOW YOURSELF

SELF-CARE REFERS TO ANY ACTIVITY THAT NURTURES you and allows you to regain your center. Self-care rituals will vary from person to person, but can include pampering, taking time off, doing deep mental health work, or even make hard choices like not giving into your cravings.

SELF-CARE SHOULD BE A TOP PRIORITY, as it will help you to be the "CEO of your Body." Practicing regular self-care routines can help you strive to be your best self, be present in life, and hopefully become a shining example for others to focus on themselves in a holistic manner.

If you have trouble keeping up with your self-care routine, consider asking a friend or someone you trust to check in and help keep you accountable. Remember, practicing self-care is not being selfish; it is a necessity in order to focus, regroup, and maintain a positive mindset.

EXAMPLES OF SELF-CARE

- Participating in activities that bring you joy and warm your heart.
- Getting quality sleep.
- Making adjustments to your schedule to help manage stress levels.
- Starting your day with 10 minutes of meditation.
- Giving your face a mini facial with daily washing.
- Taking a weekly sea salt bath.
- Staying well hydrated.
- Enjoying regular massages; learn self massage or use a foam roller.
- Eating an organic diet, including home grown herbs and vegetables from your own garden.
- Supporting your neighborhood farmers market and eating locally.
- Exercising regularly, spending time outdoors (i.e. walking for an hour daily).
- Expressing emotions when needed, such as laughing, crying, loving and showing gratitude.
- Reading books for pleasure and education.
- Traveling and having new adventures.
- Budgeting time for daily journaling, goal setting, vacations and learning new skills.
- Refraining from wearing makeup on the weekend to allow your skin to breathe.
- Practicing having a connection with nature.
- Walking barefoot in nature to recenter yourself—creates spiritual grounding.
- Planning and using grocery lists and recipes to support a Clean Eating lifestyle. A home-cooked meal is more nutritious, and knowing what you are consuming down to the ingredients is very valuable.

NOTE: *The Examples of Self-Care list is not comprehensive and can be adjusted to meet the needs of each individual. Make sure to listen to your body closely—what is right for you today may be different the next day.*

STRESS CARE

YES, YOU CAN REVERSE BAD HABITS by following these suggestions and keeping in mind that life is a journey, not a destination. You can do it!

STRESS MANAGEMENT

- Plan ahead to avoid rushed feelings.
- Learn how to relax, like *really* relax.
- Get moving. Even a small amount of movement can boost moods.
- Increase your social support.
- Meditate. This will help with focus.
- Practice gratitude. A little can build positivity and go a long way.
- Gain a growth mindset.
- Do not engage in self-judgment.

STAY AS POSITIVE AS POSSIBLE— you are doing great!

TOP SUPERFOODS TO CALM NERVES

THESE CAN KEEP YOUR CALMNESS AND SATIETY in check. Enjoy!

1. Dark green leafy vegetables are high in folate, which stimulates the serotonin and dopamine neurotransmitters to fight any onset of depression and stress.

2. Fermented foods, such as kombucha tea, are great for the vagus nerve that sends soothing signals to the brain

3. Omega-3 oils act like a soothing coat for your nervous system.

4. Blueberries and blackberries contain anthocyanins that help the brain make dopamine. Blueberries also help in the production of white blood cells to boost the immune system.

5. Pistachios help to dilate arteries for less vascular restriction, thus decreasing the stress on the heart.

6. Dark chocolate contains anandamide which is a neurotransmitter that helps to prevent depression.

7. Avocados contain minerals, vitamins, and healthy fat that create satiation and control blood sugar.

"Once we believe in ourselves, we can risk curiosity, wonder, spontaneous delight, or any experience that reveals the human spirit."

-e. e. cummings

IDEAL ADVICE

FOR LONGEVITY & HEALTH

- Spend time in nature.
- Drink more water.
- Eat hot peppers.
- Exercise.
- Practice Intermittent Fasting.
- Cook with natural ingredients.
- Keep moving during and after working hours.
- Limit time spent watching TV.
- Spend time with friends.
- Work on having healthy relationships.
- Be a lifelong learner.
- Employ breathing exercises.
- Read.
- Volunteer for good causes.
- Pursue a spiritual practice.
- Hum a melody to stimulate your vagus nerve.
- Listen to music. Dance a lot.
- Find work you love.
- Create joy whenever you can and wherever you go!

SKIN CARE

FIRST, DO YOURSELF A DELIGHT and purchase a dry skin brush. Dry skin brushing is great for detoxing and stimulating the lymph—especially first thing in the morning!

SUPPORTING SKIN DURING WEIGHT LOSS

AS WE AGE, COLLAGEN LEVELS DECREASE and skin often loses its elasticity. Use supplements like vitamin C, zinc, foods containing silica, and omega-3's during and after weight loss as they help the skin become more elastic. Also integrate the following suggestions into your routine.

- Refrain from dehydrating activities, like drinking alcohol.
- Drink at least 3 liters to 1 gallon of water a day (especially if you want to lose weight and become more active).
- Smoking and alcohol are prohibited because they decrease the elasticity of your skin.
- Build muscle through weight training, both during and after weight loss.
- Do push ups, triceps dips, bent over barbell rows, and more weights. As you are progressing, increase resistance during exercises with different intensities (if you are using therabands, the thicker the band, the more resistance).

EXERCISE IS SO IMPORTANT! LET'S DISCOVER SOME EASY SUGGESTIONS IN THE NEXT SECTION. . .

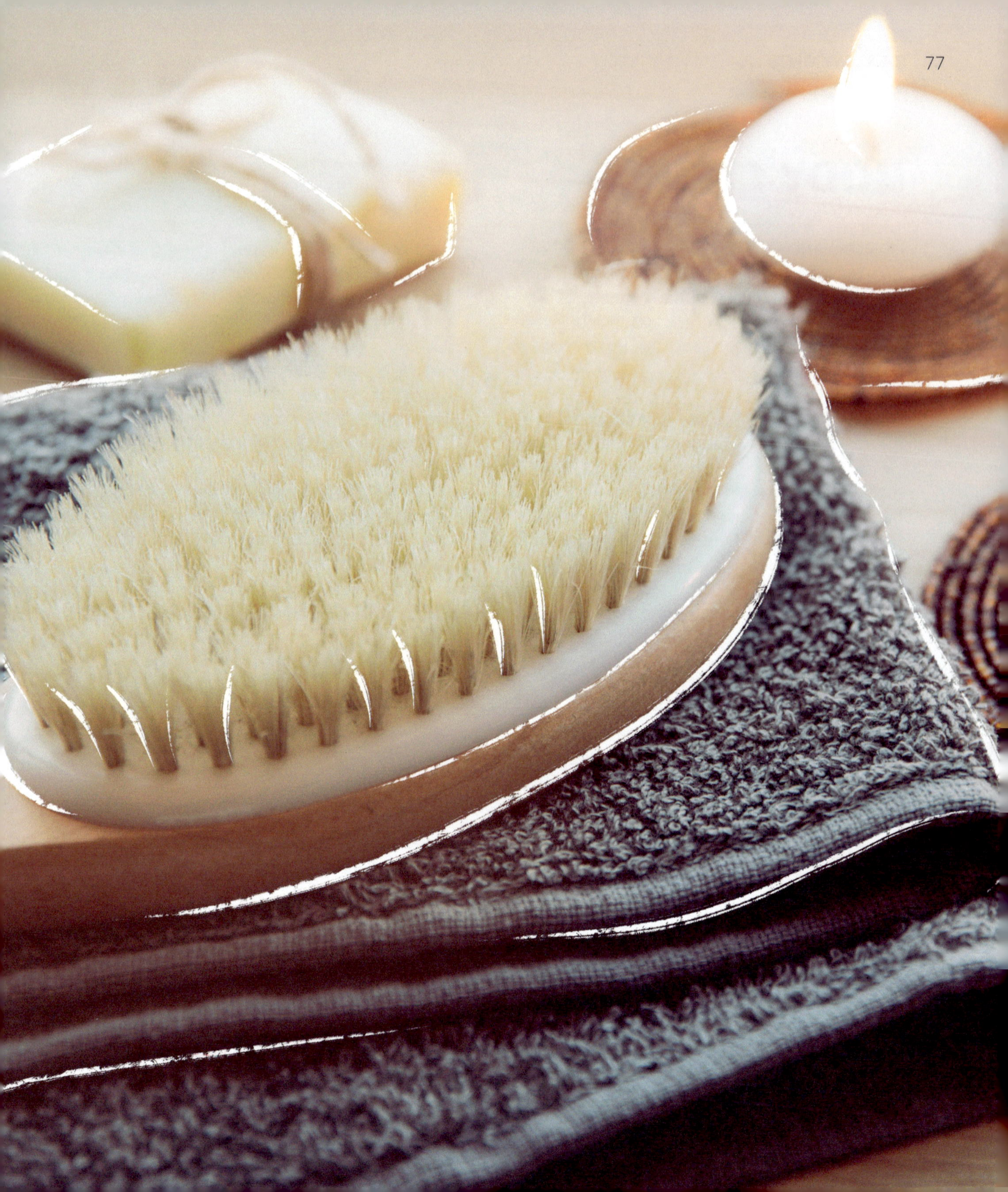

BODY CARE

EXERCISE AND PHYSICAL ACTIVITY ARE GREAT ways to feel better overall, boost your immune system, and have fun! Even small amounts of physical activity are helpful and accumulated activity throughout the day will add up to provide health benefits.

VERY EASY EXERCISES can go a long way to maintain one ideal weight or secure your next ideal weight! For me, I do free weight lifting for about 5 minutes every morning after I wake up. Besides 2-3 hours of walking on the weekends, I walk up and down 16 stairs in my house several times until my heart rate increases.

Any exercises that cause pain or bring about significant or new pain should be terminated.

DO NOT FORGET PROPER BREATHING when doing exercise. Some of the exercises might be challenging for you, but are not meant to cause excessive and out-of-proportion pain. I recommend consulting with your physician before beginning a new exercise regimen.

RECOMMENDATIONS *FROM THE DEPARTMENT OF HEALTH AND HUMAN SERVICES*

The following exercises are suggested here for most adults with stable health.

- At least 150 minutes a week of moderate activity, 75 minutes a week of vigorous aerobic activity, or a combination of moderate and vigorous activity. Guidelines suggest that you spread out your exercise activities throughout the week. Examples include: running, walking, or swimming.
- Strength training exercises for all major muscle groups at least two times a week. Examples include lifting free weights, using weight machines, or doing body weight training.
- If you want to lose weight or meet specific fitness goals, you may need to increase your moderate aerobic activity to 300 minutes or more a week.

BENEFITS OF PHYSICAL ACTIVITY

- Strengthens the immune system.
- Helps to maintain a healthy BMI.
- Improves perfusion (blood flow) to organs throughout the body.
- Increases longevity.
- Reduces the risk of certain cancers.
- Decreases the risks of many chronic illnesses, including metabolic syndrome, high blood pressure, and type 2 diabetes.
- Promotes sexual wellness.
- Improves sleep.

WHAT TO EAT DURING TRAINING

AS YOU START TO EXERCISE, you might need more protein and fat, particularly to help build muscle and burn fuel before, during, and after workouts.

PRE-WORKOUT FOOD CHOICES:

- green smoothie
- banana with almond butter
- multigrain crackers with hummus
- oatmeal with berries
- apples and walnuts

POST-WORKOUT FOOD IDEAS:

- salad with roasted chickpeas, extra virgin olive oil, and vinegar
- quinoa with blackberries and pecans
- multigrain bread with almond butter and honey
- vegetable omelet
- brown rice with black beans and avocado
- tempeh with sautéed veggies

Exercise does not have to be all or nothing. Most activities will release endorphins, also loosely referred to as "happy hormone."

These increased endorphins can help you start your day off in a different and positive manner. You do not necessarily need a certain routine or workout plan. Just start moving your body. Dance around your bedroom, park your car as far away from the entrance of the grocery store or mall, and use the stairs as often as you can.

NOTE: *Although exercise is great for a healthier body, if you are planning on having a weight loss outcome from exercise only, you would have to exercise vigorously daily. Count calories based on the numbers from page 80 to assess the number of calories you want to burn and how many hours you want to spend exercising.*

EXERCISES = CALORIES BURNED

THIS LIST SHOULD GIVE YOU A SENSE of how many calories are burned during common exercises. Numbers are approximate, as they depend on weight and intensity level.

30 MIN. OF EXERCISE:	=	CALORIES BURNED:
weight lifting	=	112
hatha yoga	=	149
walking	=	167
dancing	=	205
aerobics	=	260
jogging	=	298
elliptical	=	335
swimming	=	372
spinning	=	391

HOW TO SHAPE UP

CORE SETTING AND ABDOMINAL BREATHING, or stomach vacuuming is a breathing technique that activates and strengthens the transversus abdominis, which helps strengthen the anterior and lateral abdominal wall.

NOTE: *If you have an inguinal hernia, avoid this exercise, also make sure you perform this exercise on an empty stomach.*

TONING THE CORE

- Start by lying supine on the floor, while keeping your arms parallel to your body.
- Both knees should be bent, with both feet flat on the ground.
- Slowly exhale until you feel there is no more air left inside your lungs.
- Draw your belly button inwards and hold your breath for 15 seconds.
- After 15 seconds, slowly exhale again and repeat after returning to the starting point.

TONING THE THIGHS

I recommend repetitions of 15 each, at least 3 times a week.

- Long duration cardio (jogging/running, elliptical).
- Intense cardio.
- Lunges.
- Squats (side, froggy, jump).
- Leg scissors.
- Jumping jacks.
- Single-leg circles.
- Side leg lifts.

TONING THE BUTTOCKS

Do these exercises with or without weight.

- Ski squats.
- Butt bridges.
- Single leg raises.
- Lunges
- Squat hold (with 20-30 second holds).
- Squat pulses.
- Jump squats.
- Pop squats.

FLATTENING THE BELLY

Do these 3-5 times a week.

- Seated opposite elbow to knee crunches.
- Seated alternating knee-to-chest crunches.
- Seated double knee lift crunches.
- Supine V-holds.

IDEAL ADVICE

I recommend doing these exercises in 10-15 repetitions, at least 3 times a week.

Enjoy moving—and just do your best!

AN IDEAL DAY IN YOUR IDEAL WEIGHTS WELLNESS LIFESTYLE

TO START YOUR NEW ROUTINE, calculate your BMR and BMI (see pages 26-27) to find your suggested caloric intake. With that information, follow this protocol for two weeks using the grocery list and recipes here to meet the calories needed. Remember my main goal is not to promote weight loss in a hurry but to change your lifestyle so you can maintain weight loss for good. For a jump-start, or for maintenance, please fast intermittently. The eating times here demonstrate an Intermittent Fasting schedule. Enjoy the new and improved YOU!

MORNING

7:00 AM

UPON WAKING, write down what you are grateful for. This will create a beneficial framework for your day. Then, dry skin brush. This is a great way to move your lymph and wake yourself up!

Remember, do not weigh yourself every day. Only weigh yourself once a week to ensure you are heading in the right direction. Rely on your clothes to help you keep track (as you lose weight, they will feel looser).

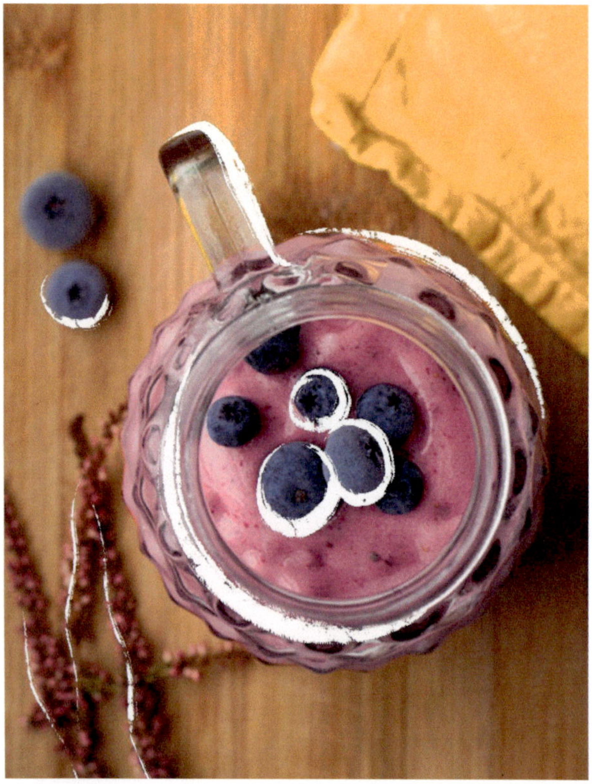

7:30-8:00 AM

MEDITATE OR DO POSITIVE AFFIRMATIONS

I am healthy. I am safe. I embrace change. I make good food decisions. I lose weight with ease. I make Clean Eating decisions. I trust my body processes. I obtain my ideal weight with grace and maintain it.

8:00-11:00 AM

DRINK A LOT OF WATER, coffee or tea. Go to work, a walk, do meal prep, tackle a project, or enjoy some food shopping.

BREAK-THE-FAST

11:00 AM–12:00 PM

BERRY BANANA SMOOTHIE

Ingredients

4 scoops of vanilla, plant based protein powder
2 cups (8-12 oz.) of milk (unsweetened almond or coconut)
1 small fresh or 1 frozen banana, sliced
1 cup fresh or frozen strawberries
1 cup fresh or frozen blueberries
1 cup of ice (in case you are using fresh fruits)

Instructions

Add all the ingredients to the blender. . .pour, sip, and salute!

Prep time = 5 minutes
Serves 2
Calories per serving : 300

AFTERNOON

GROCERY SHOPPING

IT IS STRONGLY RECOMMENDED to use organic foods when available. (Numbers in the parenthesis pertain to two weeks supply of grocery shopping.) This grocery list contains anti-inflammatory healthy foods, so you may use it as long as you wish.

Also, refer to page 19 for lists of what foods promote satiety and weight loss.

VEGETABLES:

- avocado (not to exceed 10 in 2 weeks)
- bell peppers (not to exceed 10 in 2 weeks)
- cauliflower heads (5)
- carrots (36 oz.)
- celery bunches (3)
- frozen green peas (3 bags)
- spinach bunches (9)
- red onions (8)
- yellow onions (16)
- vegetable broth or stock (1 gal.)
- spaghetti squash (3)
- jalapenos (7)
- cucumbers (2)
- roma tomatoes (8)
- cherry tomatoes (3)
- jicama (2)
- sweet potatoes (4 lb.)
- fresh tomatoes, seeded (4 lb.)
- tomato paste (2 cans)
- diced mild green chilies (4, 4 oz.)
- white mushrooms (4 pkg.)
- zucchini (2)
- black olives
- parsnip (2)

HERBS AND SPICES:

- cinnamon
- nutmeg
- pure vanilla extract
- cocoa powder (unsweetened)
- fresh thyme
- fresh rosemary
- fresh ginger
- fresh garlic
- fresh parsley
- fresh basil
- fresh oregano
- fresh cilantro
- dried bay leaf
- paprika
- black pepper
- cumin
- pink himalayan salt
- chives
- mint
- crushed red peppers
- peppercorns
- worcestershire sauce
- cardamom powder
- cayenne pepper

NUTS AND SEEDS:

- sliced almonds (1 pkg., raw)
- chia seeds (12 Tbsp.)

GRAINS:

- quinoa
- rice cakes

FRUITS:

- bananas (2)
- any fresh berries (8 oz.)
- lemons (4)
- limes (7)
- mango (2)
- peaches (6)
- raisins (1 box)
- fresh strawberries (3 pt., 6 cups)
- frozen strawberries (3 pkg.)

- frozen blueberries (3 pkg.)
- frozen peaches (2, 15 oz. pkg.)
- cantaloupe (1)

OILS AND DRESSINGS:

- apple cider vinegar (1 btl.)
- balsamic vinegar (1 btl.)
- olive oil
- avocado oil

BEANS:

- 16 cups of cooked black beans
- 8 cups of cooked garbanzo beans
- red lentils (2 pkg.)

MEAT REPLACEMENTS:

- tempeh
- seitan
- all beans
- lentils
- edamame
- pasta (plant-based)

MISCELLANEOUS:

- almond or hazelnut butter
- almond / coconut milk (2 gal., 256 oz.)
- stevia (optional)

SAMPLES OF VEGAN/VEGETARIAN SNACKS

CARBOHYDRATES:

- gluten-free bread (1 pc.) sprouted-grain bread or gluten-free tortilla (1 pc.)
- 1 slice of Ezekiel bread
- ½ cup of cooked steel oatmeal, beans, organic brown or wild rice
- ¼ cup hummus

FATS:

- 1 handful of raw, (preferably soaked) almonds or walnuts, or
- 1 handful of unsalted nuts, such as pecans and pistachio
- 1 Tbsp. of almond butterl
- 1 Tbsp. hummus

PROTEINS:

- 2-3 Tbsp. of chia / hemp / ground flax seeds
- hemp seeds (eaten cold)
- cooked mushrooms (unlimited)
- quinoa

NOTE: *Remember to pay attention to portion size. Please refer to the BMR calculation section and proceed accordingly.*

LUNCH

2:00-3:00 PM

> **NOTE:** *Take probiotics before eating! Also, know that most kinds need constant refrigeration.*

AVOCADO STRAWBERRY SPINACH SALAD

Ingredients

4 cups fresh baby spinach
2 Tbsp. of avocado oil
2 Tbsp. balsamic vinegar
½ tsp. fresh lemon juice
½ avocado, pitted and diced
¼ small red onion, thin-sliced
½ pint fresh strawberries, hulled and sliced
1 cup raw almonds, sliced

Instructions

1. Pour avocado oil, balsamic vinegar, and lemon juice together in a small bowl. Whisk to mix thoroughly. Set aside.
2. Mix spinach, strawberries, avocados, onions, and almonds together in a salad bowl.
3. Top with desired amount of vinaigrette.

Prep time = 10 minutes
Serves 2
Calories per serving: 230

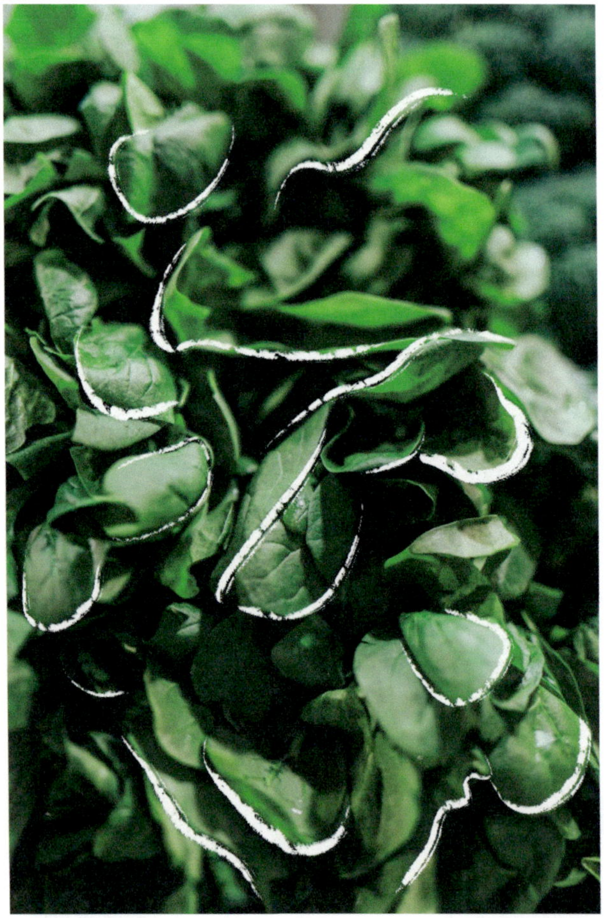

3:00-6:00 PM

WORK, WALK OR EXERCISE

SPICY BEAN SOUP

Ingredients

2 Tbsp. avocado oil
2 medium yellow onions, chopped
2 cloves garlic, minced
¼ cup green bell pepper, chopped
1 jalapeno, seeded
1tsp. chili powder
1 tsp. cumin
¼ tsp. thyme
4 cups of cooked black beans, drained
1 4 oz. can of diced mild green chilies
16 oz. organic vegetable broth
1 lime, juiced
¼ cup fresh cilantro, chopped

Instructions

1. Heat oil in a pot over medium-high heat. Add onions, garlic, green chilies, bell peppers and jalapenos. Sauté until onions are translucent, about 5 minutes.
2. Add beans, broth, chili powder, cumin and thyme.
3. Reduce heat to medium-low; cover and simmer until flavors blend, about 15 minutes.
4. Puree soup in batches in a blender and return it to the pot.
5. Add lime and cilantro to garnish.

Cooking time = 20 minutes
Serves 4
Calories per serving: 250-300

> ***NOTE:*** *Remember to take supplements with food or juice (45 minutes after your meal) for better absorption.*

EVENING

6:00-7:00 PM

DINNER OPTION # 1

BEANS AND QUINOA STUFFED PEPPERS

Ingredients

1 Tbsp. avocado oil
½ medium onion, chopped
1 stalk celery, chopped
1 Tbsp. of cumin
1 clove garlic, crushed
5 oz. spinach, fresh or frozen
2 fresh tomatoes, seeded
½ cup quinoa
¾ cup carrots, peeled and grated
½ tsp. of pink Himalayan salt
2 large bell peppers, cut in half with ribs and seeds removed
2 cups of cooked black beans, drained
1 cup of water
Optional: 1 tsp. of jalapeno peppers, seeded and chopped

Instructions

1. Heat oil in a saucepan over medium heat.
2. Add onion and celery. Cook until onion is translucent (about 5 minutes).
3. Add cumin and garlic and saute for 1 minute.
4. Stir in spinach and tomatoes, saving the liquid from the tomatoes. Cook for 5 minutes until most liquid has evaporated.
5. Mix in black beans, quinoa, carrots, hot peppers, salt, and the water. Cover and bring to a boil.
6. Preheat the oven to 375 degrees Fahrenheit.
7. Reduce heat to low. Simmer for 20 minutes, until quinoa is tender.
8. Pour the liquid from the tomatoes into the bottom of the glass baking dish.
9. Fill in each bell pepper half with ¾ cup quinoa mix and place in a baking dish. Cover with foil, and bake for 1 hour.
10. Uncover and bake for an additional 15 minutes, until tops of peppers are browned.
11. Let stand for 5 minutes and serve.

Cooking time = 2 hours
Serves 2
Calories per serving 250

DINNER OPTION #2

ROASTED VEGETABLE TACOS WITH CHIPOTLE HUMMUS

Ingredients

For the roasted vegetables:

2 medium onions, chopped
2 large zucchini, chopped
2 red peppers chopped
2 Tbsp. avocado oil
1 tsp. dry oregano
½ tsp. Himalayan salt

For the hummus:

1 ½ cup cooked chickpeas
1 cup tahini
½ cup of water
¼ cup of lime juice
1 ½ canned chipotle en adobo, diced
1 Tbsp. avocado oil
6 gluten-free or low-carb tortillas
Optional: toppings of diced avocado, chopped cilantro

Instructions

1. Preheat the oven to 400 degrees Fahrenheit. Cover a large baking sheet with parchment paper.
2. Place the avocado oil, red pepper, onions, oregano, zucchini, and salt in a large bowl and toss well. Transfer to the lined baking sheet and bake for 35 minutes. Bake longer if you want your vegetables more tender.
3. Place all the ingredients for chipotle hummus in a food processor and process until creamy. Put aside (or refrigerate until ready to use).
4. To assemble the tacos, spread hummus on each tortilla and top with vegetables.
5. If desired, sprinkle chopped cilantro and dice avocado on top of the tortillas and enjoy!

Cooking time = 35 minutes
Serves 8
Calories per serving: 240

DESERT

7:00 PM

CREAMY COCOA PUDDING

Ingredients

2 medium avocados, peeled, pitted, and diced
1/3 cup cocoa powder
1 cup almond or coconut milk beverage
1 tsp. cinnamon
2 tsp. vanilla extract
¼ cup frozen blueberries and strawberries mix
½ tsp. pink Himalayan salt
1 Tbsp. slivered almonds
Stevia to taste (optional)

Instructions

1. Place all ingredients into a blender and puree until creamy.
2. Chill in the refrigerator for 2-3 hours.

Prep. time = 5 minutes
Total time = 3 hours
Serves 4
Calories per serving: 130

7:15 PM

TAKE SUPPLEMENTS

8:00 PM

TURN OFF SCREENS

BEDTIME

9:00 PM

START SLEEP ROUTINE

Brush your teeth after dinner to help avoid unnecessary snacking. Write down what you are proud of yourself for, each and every day. Enjoy the small wins. This will create confidence and the furthering of your dreams!

Tomorrow is another day on your journey to ideal health. Keep at it!

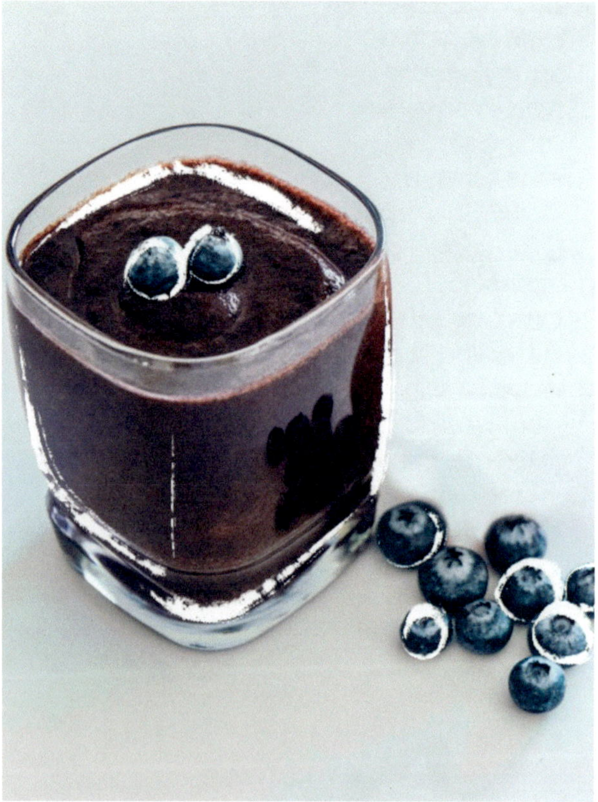

RAICINN CHIA DELIGHT

Prep this for tomorrow's breakfast.

Ingredients

1 cup milk (unsweetened almond or coconut)
3 Tbsp. of chia seeds
1 tsp.. ground cinnamon
1 tsp. pure vanilla extract
2 Tbsp. raisins

Instructions

1. In a bowl, mix all ingredients except raisins. Stir.
2. Cover and refrigerate overnight.
3. In the morning, top it off with raisins.

Prep time = 5 minutes
Total time = 8 hours
Serves 2
Calories per serving: 230

AFTERWORD

CONGRATULATIONS—You are well on your weight-loss journey! I hope the application of Ideal Weights is as enjoyable to you as it was for me, and that you embrace gaining a new healthy lifestyle.

The Ideal Weights approach is a guide that helps understand the Body-Mind Connection with various foods and aims to avoid the typical "yo-yo" dieting approach. "Yo-yo" dieting is harmful to the body, creating a routine that can often be easily adopted, but more easily abandoned.

Conversely, my Ideal Weights protocol focuses on continuity rather than a quick fix.

Now, I want to share a story with you that is not a typical "before and after" tale. It is more about reaching one ideal weight, and then achieving the next ideal weight that you desire.

This first picture was taken in 2015. Here I am, healthier than I had ever been—with extra energy!

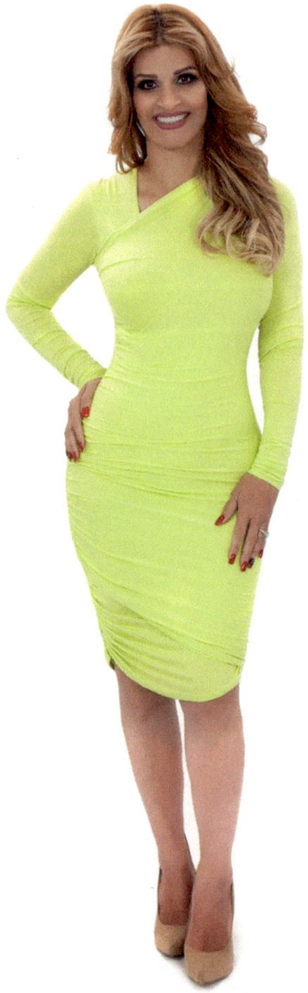

2015

Feeling this good motivated me to keep it up. So I kept the same yellow dress (from when I was featured on the front cover of the *Calabasas Times* magazine) to see if my newfound health regimen would really work long term.

And voila! This second picture was taken in February of 2020.

The dress still fits! Especially since I became ovo-vegan it was easier to keep my size and shape. Eating plant-based foods mindfully, fasting intermittently, removing toxins, and taking vitamin D and supplementation works. These pictures are the proof.

If you commit, the dress will fit!

YOURS IN HEALTH,

DR. MAHNAZ AZIM, DC

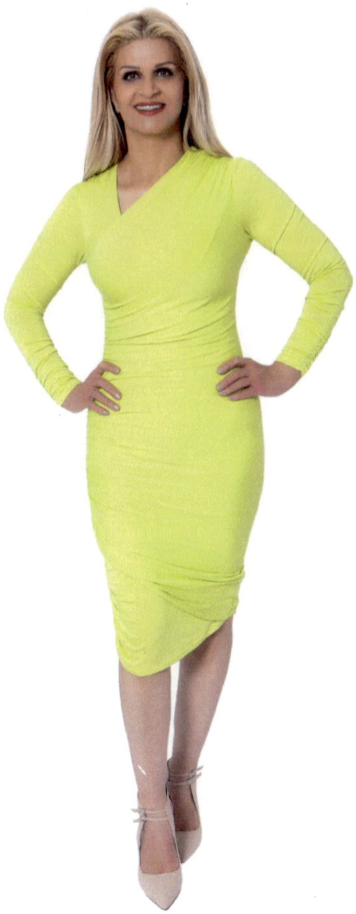

2020

IDEAL WEIGHTS

To find out more, visit idealweights.com

Made in the USA
Monee, IL
05 November 2026

67385918R00064